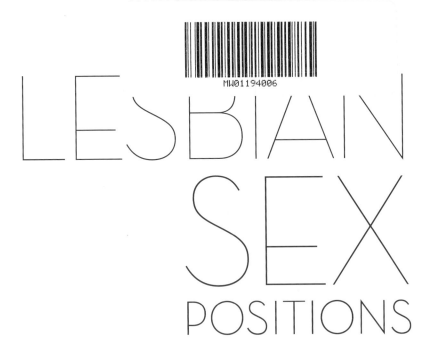

LESBIAN
SEX
POSITIONS

LESBIAN SEX POSITIONS

100 Passionate Positions from Intimate and Sensual to Wild and Naughty

Shanna Katz, MEd, ACS

Amorata Press

Published by:
AMORATA PRESS,
an imprint of Ulysses Press
P.O. Box 3440
Berkeley, CA 94703
www.amoratapress.com

A Hollan Publishing, Inc. Concept

ISBN13: 978-1-61243-229-8
Library of Congress Control Number: 2013938524

Printed in Korea by WE SP through Four Colour Print Group

10 9 8 7 6 5 4 3 2 1

Acquisitions Editor: Keith Riegert
Managing Editor: Claire Chun
Editor: Paula Dragosh
Proofreader: Elyce Berrigan-Dunlop
Interior design: Jake Flaherty
Photography: Hollan Publishing, Inc.

CONTENTS

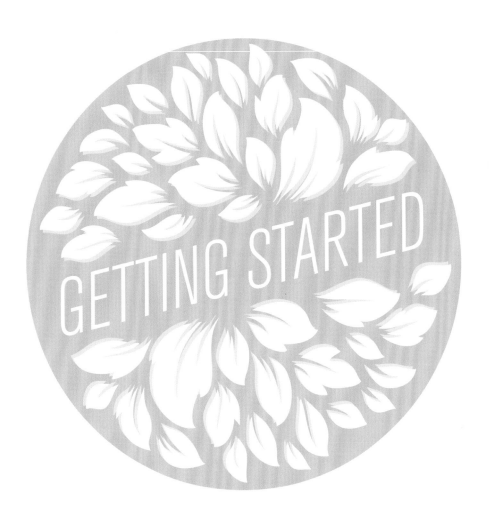

GETTING STARTED

INTRODUCTION

When I sat down to begin writing this book, I had to struggle with the question What is lesbian sex?

You can't really put orientation or identity on sexual acts. Think about it: if putting a penis in an anus is "gay sex," then what does it mean when a straight guy puts his penis in his female partner's butt? If rubbing up on someone's thigh is a sign of "lesbian sex"…then what happens when two men or a man and a woman do it? Sex isn't black and white. You might say that it is shades of gray.

For this book, let's just focus on all the exciting sexual acts that can take place between two women. This means that this book is for all women: lesbian women, bisexual women, straight women experimenting, homoflexible women, heteroflexible women, or questioning women— or any other orientation! It's for women who were assigned female at birth, women who have transitioned into their true gender, and those who aren't quite sure where they are on the gender spectrum but are turned on by what's going on over the following pages (the anatomy might be a little more diverse, but overall, the theories apply to all women). Basically, if you like women and have made it this far, this book is for you.

Sex is more than just two (or more!) bodies coming together for genital touching and orgasmic gratification. It's all of the other pieces that optimize your sexual experience. I cover many of those tools that can help you to have the sex you want, to please yourself and your partner(s), and to be a true explorer of the wonderful world of sexuality.

Communication is key to creating good sex. To truly communicate what you want and need to someone else means that you first need to understand your body and your mind, and what your wants and needs really are. Pick up on some tips and techniques to ramp-up your communication, which will result in making sure your needs are getting met and the sex is satisfying in all the ways you want it to be.

This book is for you to do with what you wish. Read it cover to cover, or hone in on the areas that interest you the most. Enjoy it, put it to good use, and relish your sexual explorations as you continue to grow as a sexual being!

ANATOMY:
What's Going On Down There?

The mons pubis is often referred to as the pubic bone, or the Mound of Venus. It's naturally covered in pubic hair (although some people will choose to trim/shave/decorate this hair). It can be fun to rub, touch, and stroke this area. Because the nerves of the clitoris actually extend under this area, many people like to have it pressed on with the palm of the hand.

In regard to labia, the Latin gets it a little wrong. In scientific terms, these lips are known as the labia majora (big lips) and labia minora (little lips). This is often incorrect. Vulvas are like snowflakes: each one is completely different. Sometimes the labia minora are larger than the labia majora, sometimes they're the same size. Let's stick with calling them inner lips and outer lips.

Outer lips come naturally with pubic hair and lie on either side of the vulva. Inner lips are thinner, hairless, and can either be tucked between the outer lips or extend beyond them. It's normal for lips to be uneven, have different coloration, etc. Nothing that a person does can change the size or length of the inner labia. Whatever size, shape, color, or length, that these inner lips are is exactly the way that they're supposed to be.

Many women like having their labia stimulated and played with, some rougher than others. Some will just enjoy gentle stroking and soft touch, others will want a little bit of pulling or maybe some nibbling.

THE CLIT

The tops of the inner lips lead up toward the top of the vulva, forming the clitoral hood, which is a cover for the actual clitoris itself. This hood is a thin covering of skin protecting the sensitive clitoris from too much stimulation before it's ready. It acts almost as an eyelid, covering up the clit from the outside world.

Some think the clitoris is just the glans below the clitoral hood. In fact, the clitoris is shaped like a wishbone and has 3- to 6-inch legs that extend below the vulva underneath the labia.

With arousal, the clitoral hood will pull back slightly, allowing more access. Many people also enjoy having oral stimulation of the lips, hood, and clitoris, whether it's licking, sucking, or gentle nibbling. Other vulva owners like the feeling of vibrators on their clitoris.

Between the clitoral glans/hood and vaginal opening is the urethra, which is where urine comes out. For those who can ejaculate during

G-spot stimulation, this is where the ejaculatory fluid comes out. Some people may enjoy having the area around the urethra (the urinary meatus) stimulated gently with a finger. Always be gentle, and only stimulate this area with clean fingers or clean toys.

THE VAGINA

The vaginal opening is filled with nerves. Lots of people like having the opening gently played with, regardless of whether anything will actually be going inside. While many vulvas naturally lubricate, some don't, and extra lube is always welcome.

Past the vaginal opening, there's the vaginal canal, or what most people just refer to as the vagina. Vaginas vary in depth; the average is 5 to 8 inches. Some can be shallower, especially if there's an inverted uterus. The majority of the sensation is in the front third of the vagina, which is why many people say that they prefer girth more than length in their partners and toys. It's also why lots of folks report that they prefer the first few strokes of being penetrated (whether by fingers, toys, or penises) because they stimulate this area. The legs of the clitoris run under the labia and hug the opening of the vaginal canal, helping provide these sensations.

The vaginal canal is capped at the end with the cervix, with a tiny opening called the os. The cervix is like a cap on the end of the vagina.

The os will open slightly to allow menstrual fluid out and may dilate to allow a baby through during birth, but otherwise, it's closed. You CANNOT lose things in the vagina. If at any point you're worried about something being "lost" in there, just relax as much as you can and gently place lubricated fingers (yours or your partner's) inside to carefully pull the item out.

KEGELS

Interested in experiencing deeper, stronger, more intense vaginal orgasms? Take a moment to squeeze your pelvic muscles. It's like you're trying to stop the flow of your urine. Then push out. Squeeze in. And repeat. Those are your PC (pubococcygeus) muscles! After working these muscles out a while, you can hold them in for a longer period of time. If you need a little extra help, try Kegel balls (meant to be worn while you walk around), Kegelcisors, or Kegel barbells.

FINDING THE G-SPOT

That brings us to the G-spot, sometimes called the urethral sponge. Named after the spot's original discoverer and proponent, Dr. Ernst Gräfenberg, the Gräfenberg spot is about 1 to 3 inches inside the vaginal canal, at the top, and feels kind of spongy or bumpy. It can usually be found either with a toy that has a nice curve or by inserting fingers into the vagina and making a "come here" motion.

The important thing to note about the G–spot is that it doesn't always exist. The G–spot is only there when the person with the vagina is incredibly aroused. Just like any other body part, people like to have this area stimulated in different ways, and while for some people the G–spot is finding the holy grail, others may find it to be just "meh" or even annoying.

Let's discuss ejaculation! Even if you weren't born with a penis, you can experience the bodily function that is ejaculation. The first important thing to know about this ejaculatory fluid: it is not pee. In case you were worried about it, you can rest easy knowing it's not, in fact, urine.

In fact, ejaculate is created in the Skene's gland, and when the G–spot is fully aroused and stimulated, sometimes this gland releases ejaculatory fluid through the urethra. It can happen at the same time as an orgasm, it can happen without an orgasm, and of course, orgasms can happen without ejaculation being part of the equation. It's all normal, fun, and fabulous. As far as the amount that comes out, it can vary between a few drops and almost half a cup. The amount released has no correlation to how aroused the woman is.

Once we hit the end of this vulvar goodness, there lies the perineum. Some people call this the "taint," others call it a pleasure zone, and more names abound. The area is filled with more nerve endings; some people find it pleasurable when stimulated.

ANAL PLAY

Upon reaching the other end of the perineum, we have arrived at the anus. While the anus is not part of the vulva itself, it contains all of its own nerves and fun tricks. Whether you and your partner want to enjoy manual stimulation of the anus with fingers, oral fun, or penetration, the anus can add a whole new dimension to your sexy playtime.

Anal tissue is incredibly delicate. Because of this, you want to make sure that you're always careful and gentle when playing with the area, both externally and internally. Also, the anus provides no natural lubricant. None. This means that it's crucial to add lube when playing with the backdoor. Check out the section on lubricants (page 252) to learn more about the different varieties of lube available for use.

You can also provide stimulation of the anal opening, which is full of nerves that will feel wonderful to many people. Some people love anal stimulation, some hate it, and many are neutral. Make sure to have that conversation about what your partner likes (and doesn't like!) before you try to stick your finger in her bottom.

THE BREASTS

The breasts can absolutely be considered their own sex organ. The larger circle in the middle of the breast is called the *areola*, and the smaller nub in the middle is the *nipple*. They come in all shapes, sizes, and colors. The size of the breasts, the areolas, and the nipples has nothing to do with the type of sensation women experience and how they like their breasts played with. Some breasts and nipples like gentle touch and pressure, like feather ticklers, fingertips, and a light lick of your tongue. Others prefer to be grabbed, groped, pulled, pinched, bitten, sucked, and more. Figure out what you like and share it with your partner for better sensation so she'll know what feels good.

TELL ME WHAT YOU WANT
(What You Really, Really Want!)
COMMUNICATION

If you read this book and put it down with only one take-home message, let that message be: Communication Is Key.

Vulvas were not built as one size fits all. Most people are often in the midst of trying to figure out what their own body likes and doesn't like, and what their own needs are. It gets more complicated because most female bodies change based on stress, the menstrual cycle, or other random things. Something that your body may love one day may feel icky a week later. Bodies are hard to figure out, even our own, yet we assume that our partners will magically be able to figure out what we like at a moment's notice.

We are responsible for giving (and receiving) feedback. When something feels good, you should let your partner know. If something doesn't feel so great, it's up to you to tell your partner that it might not be the right thing for you. Not only do you have to be willing to communicate things that are relevant to your body, but you also have to be willing to solicit feedback from your partner.

Communicating doesn't have to involve hours of conversation, contracts, and paperwork. Nor should it be a one-time thing (unless it's a one-time fling). Even if you're just hooking up in a club bathroom, you can still communicate. It's still communication, even though it's quick. If you're in a longer-term relationship, then you should be constantly communicating. If you work communication into your regular interactions, there's a lot less pressure and stress to "fix" something right away.

Keep in mind that communication doesn't always have to be direct verbal contact. Figure out which types of communication work best for you and which work for your partner. It's possible that one of you needs the most direct communication possible. It's equally possible that one of you might prefer certain levels of gasping and groaning, or pulling hair, pinching nipples, or placing your partner's hand on top of your own to guide you to the right areas and amounts of pressure.

Some of us might have hang-ups from previous people we dated; former relationships and ex-partners can definitely influence our communication style. Keep working at it; it takes two to tango, and also at least two to communicate. Remember that the way you like to be communicated with might not be the same way that your partner wants to receive communication.

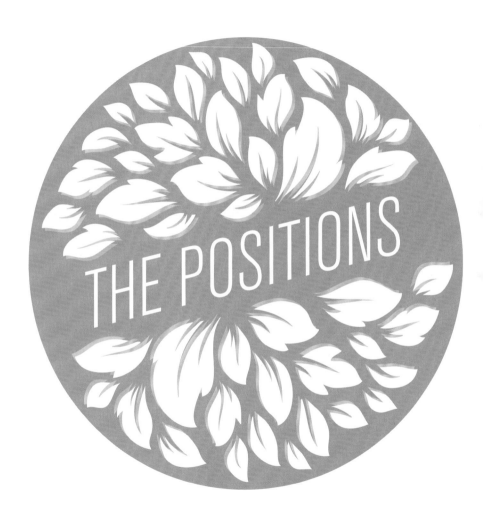

GENTLE TOUCH

For some, manual stimulation is foreplay or part of another sexual activity, but when done well, fingering, finger fucking, handiwork, or whatever you'd like to call it can be pretty incredible by itself. The key to being good with your fingers is remembering that you're using them to give your partner pleasure. Some women can have upward of a dozen orgasms simply with the proper stimulation by their partner's fingers. Start out slowly, and work your way up to more stimulation as you work her into a frenzy.

How can you be sure of being safe during this wonderful handiwork? Bring on the gloves! They're easy to find. Most grocery stores and drugstores have them, but if you want fun colors, look online for gloves marketed to tattoo artists and doctor's offices. You can find them in almost every color of the rainbow, even black. Why are gloves important? Not only can sexually transmitted infections (STIs) be transmitted from person to person via vaginal fluid on hands, but gloves are awesome for many reasons—they help prevent the person being pleasured from getting small cuts and tears in and around her vagina from long fingernails and, since vaginal fluid tends to be slightly acidic, gloves can protect hands from feeling a slight stinging in small cuts and rough patches.

If you want to be the best that you can be in the realm of fabulous fingering, you have to communicate with your partner to understand her likes. Different positions are better for different needs; the better you get to know her body, the better the sex will be. Remember to communicate, have fun, and that practice makes perfect. The more you get it on, the better it'll be the next time because you'll have learned just a bit more about each other's bodies and what gets you going. The more you know, the more incredibly satisfying your sexual encounters can be!

Getting Things Rolling

Most of us don't go from 0 to 60 in seconds flat; it is important for both partners to get the right amount of warm-up before you delve into anything and everything else. Slowly running your hands over her body, kissing her deeply, and just preparing each other for what is yet to come (pun intended) is just as important as any of the other positions in this book. Don't rush things unless you both are ready to go; savor the sensations of touch, the lusciousness of lips, and so much more!

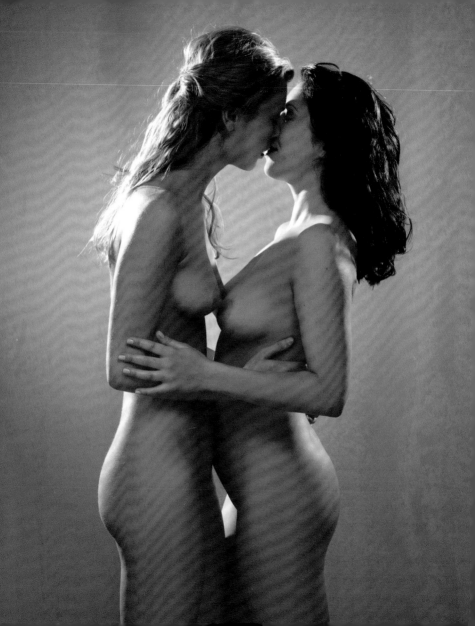

The Tempting Tease

So often we focus on the main event, whether that is fingering, oral sex, toying around, or more. However, then we miss out on the delicious delight of tantalizing and teasing someone until their nerves are heightened and they can barely take it any more. There is much to be said for slooooowly slipping a hand into your lover's panties, kissing along their bra line, licking them over their lingerie, and really revving them into gear before you even take off their clothes!

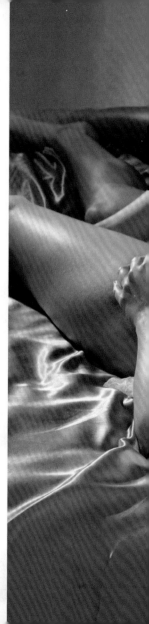

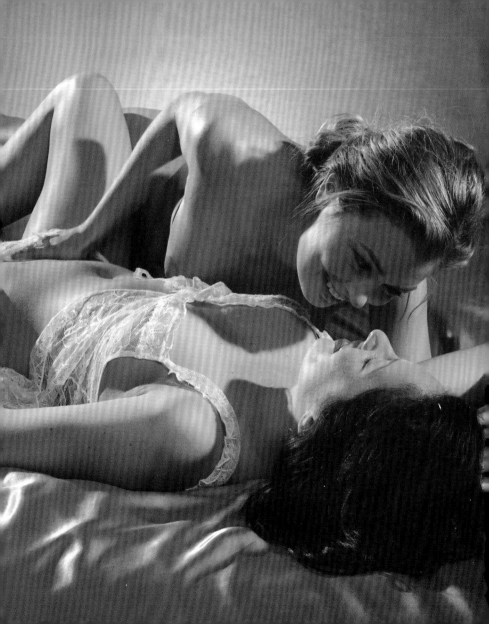

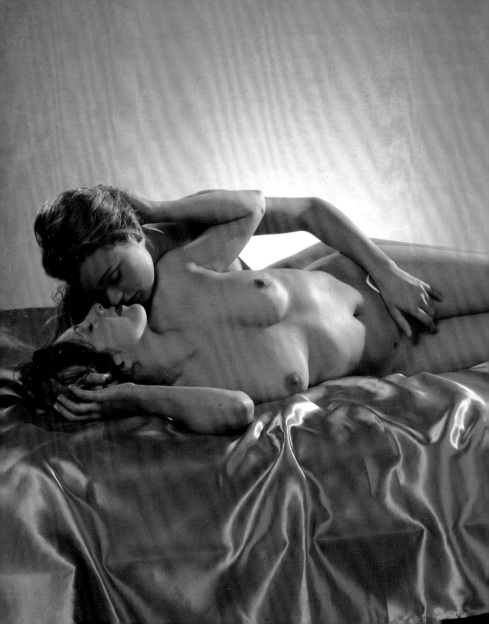

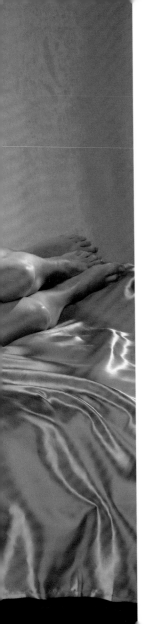

Concentric Cuddling

Both partners are lying in bed together, on their sides, spooning. The woman in back has her hand over her partner's hips and is stimulating her partner's vulva. She can also be kissing her partner's neck, playing with her nipples, and so on. The front partner can choose to use her hands to lift herself up in order to stimulate her own vulva or to use a toy to add a different dimension.

Fully Focused

The receiving partner is lying on her back, knees up and gently spread. The partner providing pleasure is sitting next to her hips, with her legs placed toward the head of the partner who is lying down. This way, she can fully focus on what she is doing to her partner's vulva, giving her waves of sensual stimulation. It's a great position for adding in some action from a sex toy and wonderful for both partners to make and keep eye contact throughout.

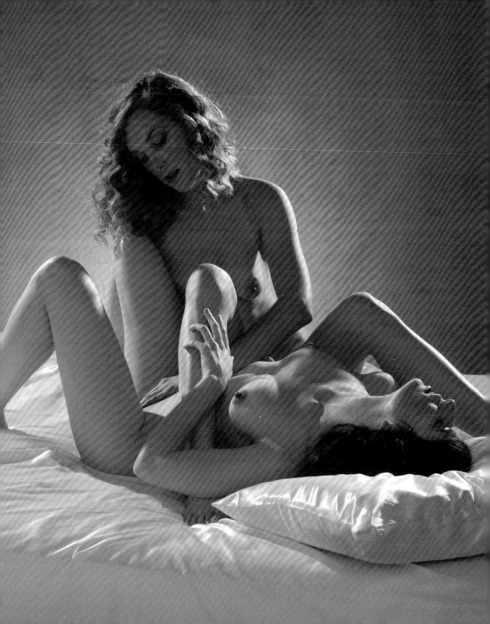

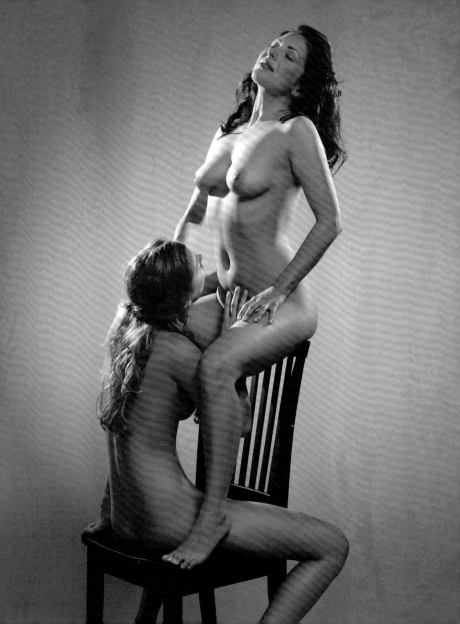

Sittin' Pretty

One partner is straddling a chair (make sure not to use a rocking chair!), while the other is sitting on the back of the chair, facing her partner, with her feet planted on the sitting part of the chair. The partner who is higher up is able to open her legs and give great access right at eye level to her lover, who can play with her using her fingers or even toys, as well as reach up to stimulate nipples and more. Just be careful!

Mirror Mirror

This position is a great way to have 100 percent safer sex; the two partners are kneeling next to each other on the bed (or can be lying down if they prefer), and are both stimulating themselves. This way, both can learn about how the other prefers to be stimulated, and there is no fluid exchange, making the sex safe from transmissions of STIs while remaining incredibly visually stimulating. Toys can be used, but should not be shared unless the two individuals are fluid bound or are using safer-sex supplies.

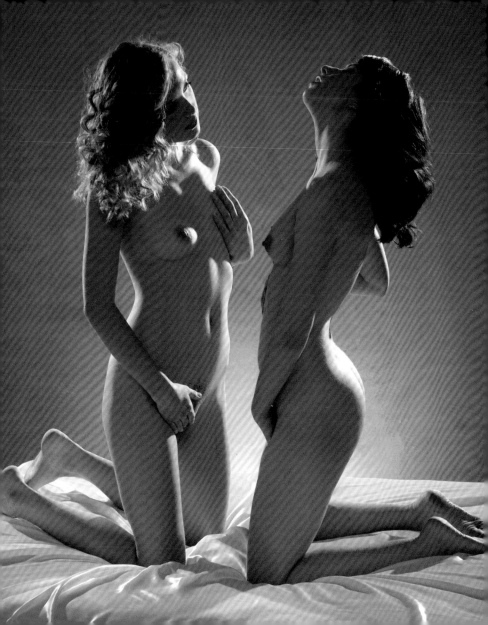

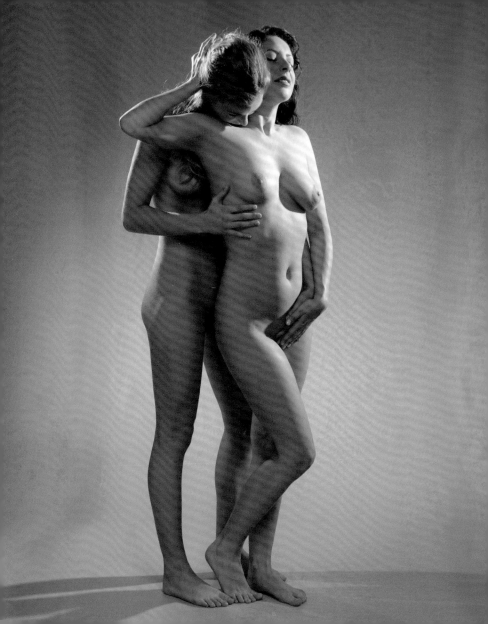

Standing Stimulation

Both partners are standing, facing the same direction. One woman is in front of the other, their bodies pressed close together. The woman in back is reaching around her partner with both hands, one stimulating the front partner's nipples and the other reaching down to stimulate the vulva. The woman in front can help out by stimulating herself or even by bringing a toy into the mix if she'd like.

All Wound Up

Both partners are sitting, facing each other, with their knees slightly bent. One woman has her legs on the outside, the other on the inside, allowing them each access to the other's genitals while still being able to support themselves with their other arm. This is a great position that allows for breast stimulation, connective eye contact, and as much kissing as they both want. It can also take place on the floor with pillows for comfort.

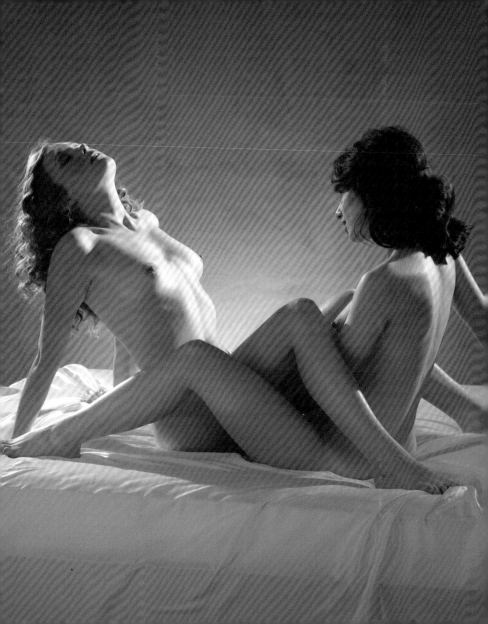

The Vitruvian Woman

One woman lies on her back on the bed, with her legs together, arms at her sides. Her partner lies on top of her, face up, and spreads her legs and arms wide. The woman on the bottom reaches around her partner to stimulate her vulva (it looks like Da Vinci's "Vitruvian Man" diagram). You can definitely add toys to this position to mix things up.

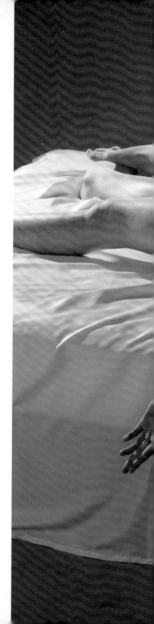

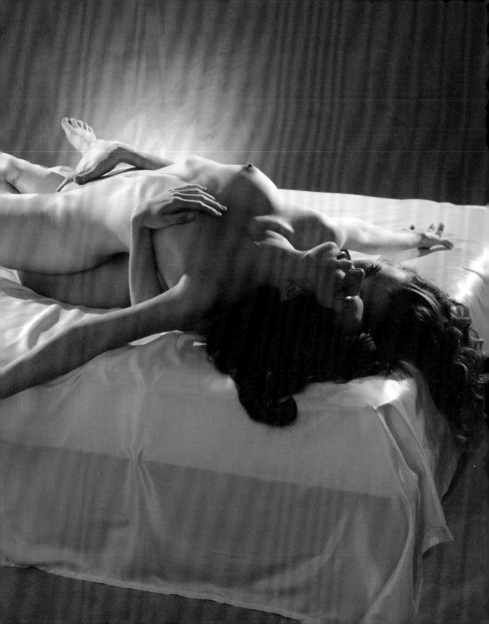

The Chairwoman

One partner is sitting in a comfortable chair facing outward while the other partner sits on her lap, facing the same direction. The woman on the chair can then reach around to stimulate her partner's breasts and vulva, while the woman in front can turn around for a kiss. One great way to use this position is while watching a hot movie or porn film, or even while whispering sweet nothings to one another.

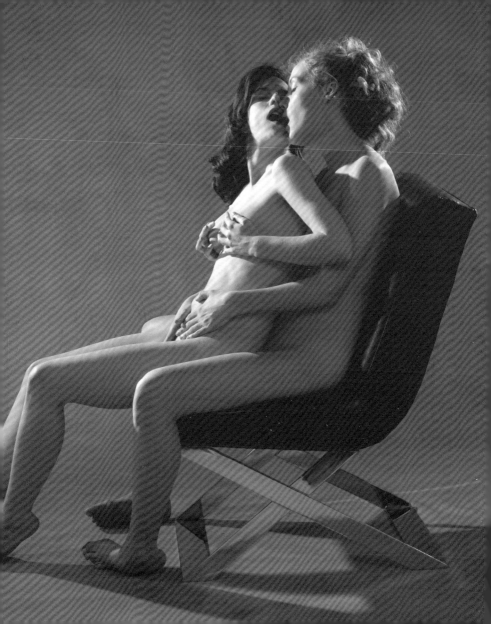

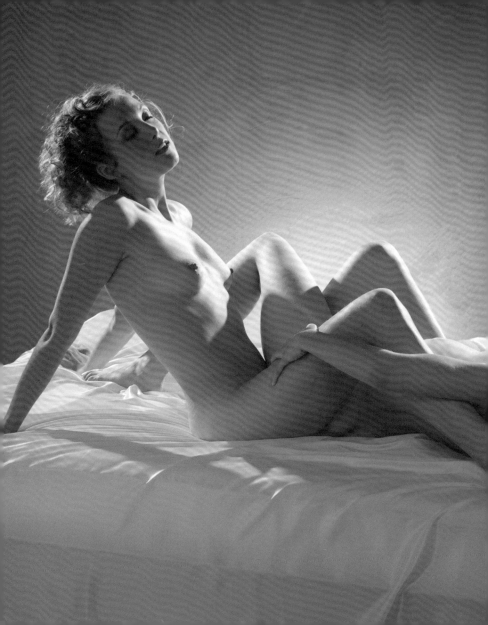

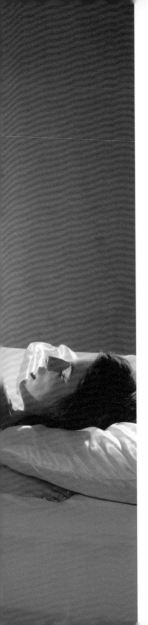

Double Desire

A position designed for partners who want to stimulate each other at the same time, this position has one woman lying down on her back (propping her up with pillows can add comfort and accessibility) while her partner lies next to her with her head and feet reversed. This way, both can stimulate their lover simultaneously, resulting in pleasure for them both.

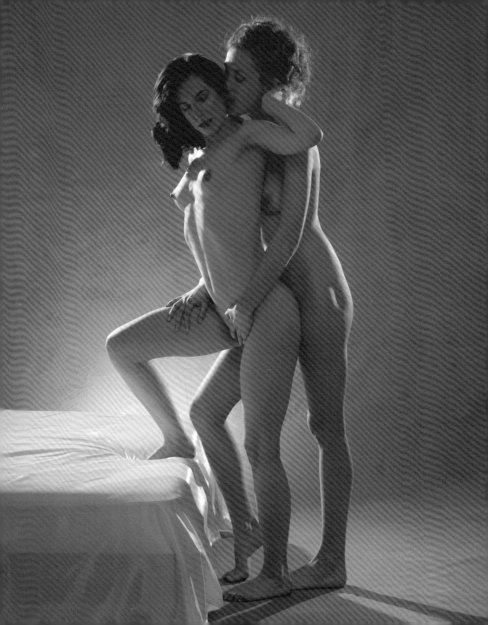

Stepping It Up

Both partners are standing by the bed, facing the same direction. The woman in front has raised one of her legs, bent at the knee, and is resting her foot on the bed (or a chair or step—whatever works best) to allow more access to her vulva. Her partner is standing behind her, helping support her with one arm around the waist and the other reaching around to stimulate her vulva, nipples, and so on. Of course, you can also involve a vibrator or dildo.

The Two-Finger Pet

The receiving woman is lying on her back on the bed with her legs spread and bent at the knees, feet flat on the bed. Her partner is lying on her stomach, with her face near her partner's vulva, putting two (or more!) fingers in her partner's vagina with one hand and stimulating her partner's clitoris with the other. You can also add vibrators and dildos to this position, depending on what feels best for you and your partner.

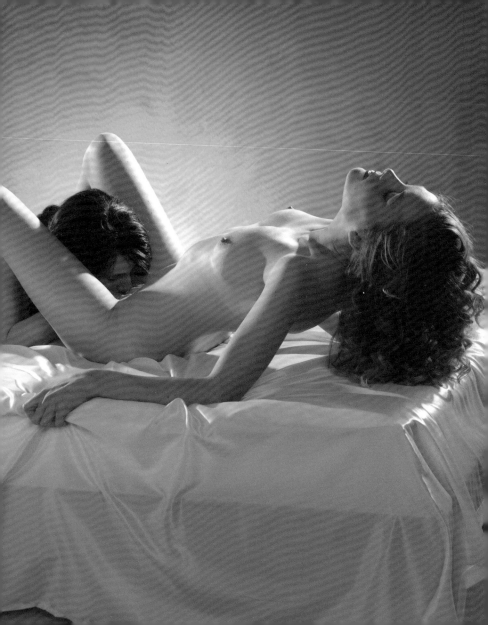

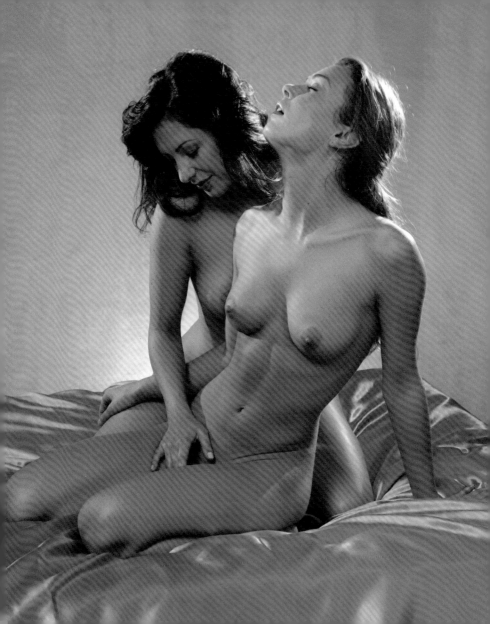

The Raunchy Reach-Around

Both partners are sitting or kneeling on the bed (or floor), both facing the same direction. The woman behind is reaching around her partner's hips, stimulating her vulva with fingers or a toy. She can use her other hand to wrap in her partner's hair or stimulate her nipples. The front partner can participate as well or just enjoy the pleasurable sensations.

The Anchor

One woman has her head and shoulders on the floor supported by pillows, with her legs reaching up. Her knees are bent, her feet are flat on the edge of the bed. This places her hips and vulva at the edge. Her partner is on the bed, either lying on her stomach or crouched on her hands and knees. She reaches down to play with her partner's vulva. She can offer penetration, or clitoral stimulation, or a combination of both.

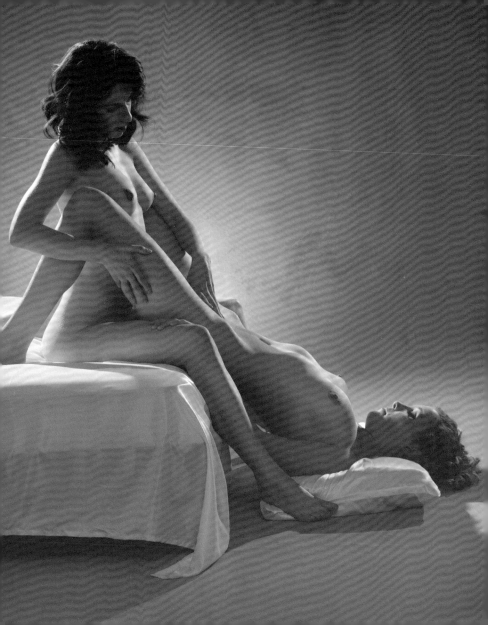

Acute Angles

The receiver lies on the bed, legs spread with her feet placed on the bed, her knees bent. Her partner is sitting (or kneeling) in front of her, between her legs, facing her. The partner sitting is stimulating her partner's vulva with her hands and can reach up to stimulate her nipples and can also use toys if she chooses. The woman on the bed can use her hands to stimulate her own nipples. Placing a pillow below her hips can help create better angles and access.

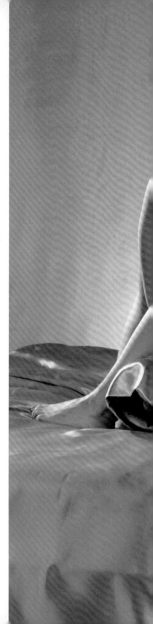

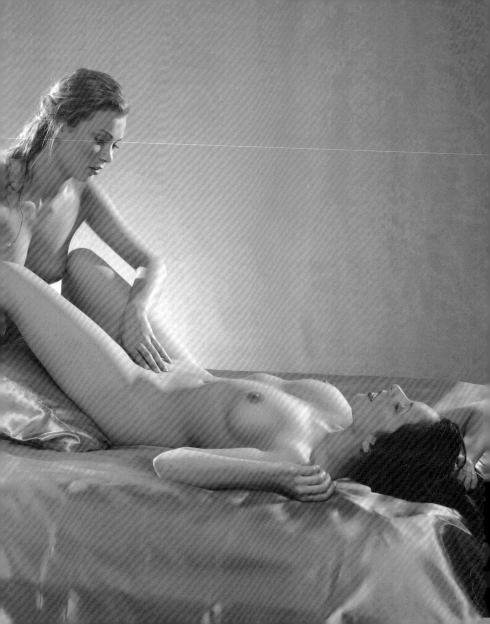

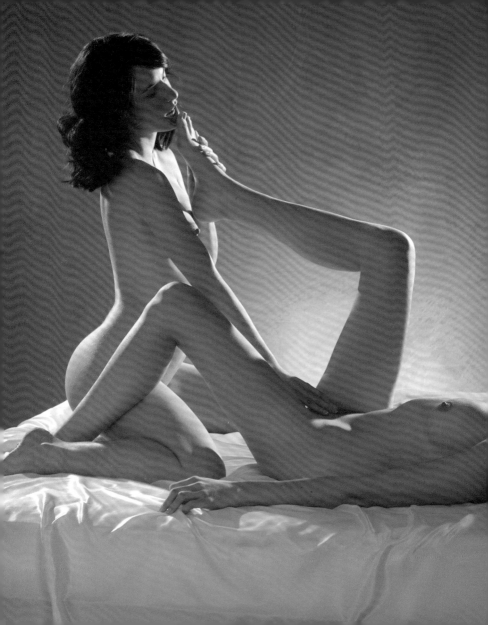

Tantalizing Toes

Ideal for those who are attracted to feet or have a foot fetish of some sort, this position has one woman lying on her back with the other kneeling between her legs. The woman on her back can offer her feet up to her partner, and the kneeling partner can stimulate her lover while also getting to enjoy her fabulous feet. Consider using pillows to raise the hips and/or head of the partner who is lying down for better angles.

Look Ma, Two Hands!

One woman is on the bed on her hands and knees, and her partner is kneeling directly behind her (she can place a pillow under her knees to cushion them if need be). The woman kneeling behind reaches between her partner's legs to penetrate her vaginally (or play with her anus or clitoris) while reaching around to stimulate her partner's nipples or pull her hair. This could be a great position for using a blindfold.

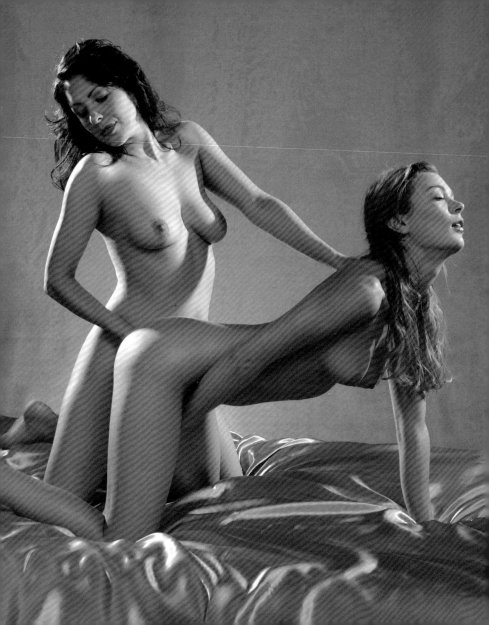

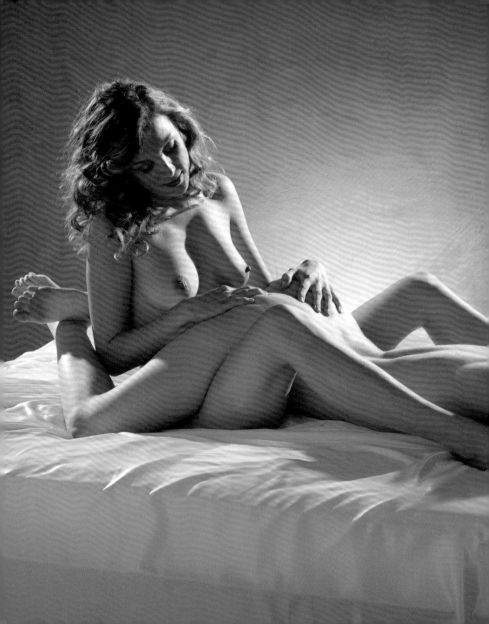

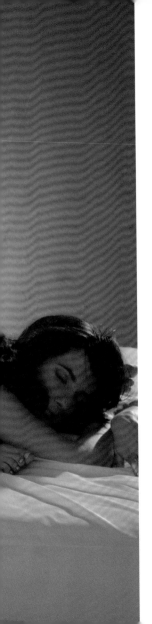

Buena Vista

A position designed for those who really love a gorgeous view of their lover's delicious backside, this allows the person giving the pleasure to have an up close and personal view of their favorite body part while getting to stimulate their partner. It is also a great position for anyone with mobility issues, as there is little to no pressure on the joints.

Up and Over

One woman is lying on her back, stimulating her own vulva, while her legs are resting on the shoulders of her partner, who is kneeling directly in front of her. Great for safer sex or when one person wants to receive kisses, touch, and stimulation all over her body while she gives herself pleasure. Also great for one partner to show the other how and where she likes to be touched as a bit of a sensual, hands-on peep show.

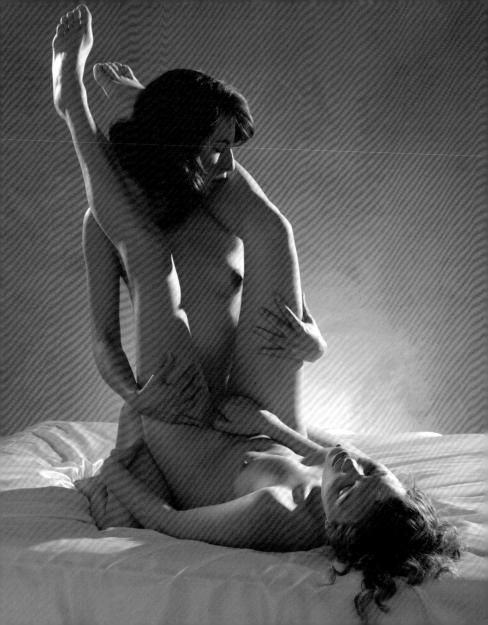

FRICTION

While of course there are many other ways women can have sex with other women, one way is through friction. "Scissoring" is a very limited term, but tribadism (which is the scientific name) and frottage (the scientific name for rubbing one part of your body against another body part sexually) are fun things that can happen between two people.

For some, playing with friction as part of sex creates tension, or warm-up during foreplay. For those who have chosen not to be traditionally sexually intimate (i.e., focusing on penetration), friction can be done with clothes on; there's no transmission of fluid and you can build on, or even change up your concept of the main course. Others view friction as the main course of their sexual time together, experiencing great pleasure and orgasms from rubbing against each other.

Like all sex, there's no right or wrong way. Do what feels good. I've provided some suggestions to get you started, but this is the time to experiment. Try wearing full clothing, just your underwear, or nothing at all. Add in chairs and other furniture to change positions. If you have multiple partners, you can add in some friction action to make sure they're getting some pleasurable attention while something else is going on. The possibilities are endless!

Sexy Scissors

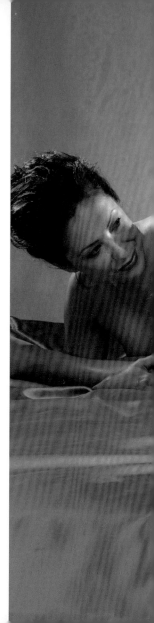

Both partners are lying on their sides, with their heads at opposite ends of the bed, their bodies facing the same direction. Their legs have slid open to allow their vulvas to touch. This is the traditional way scissoring is viewed and may be worth a try for people interested in making it happen.

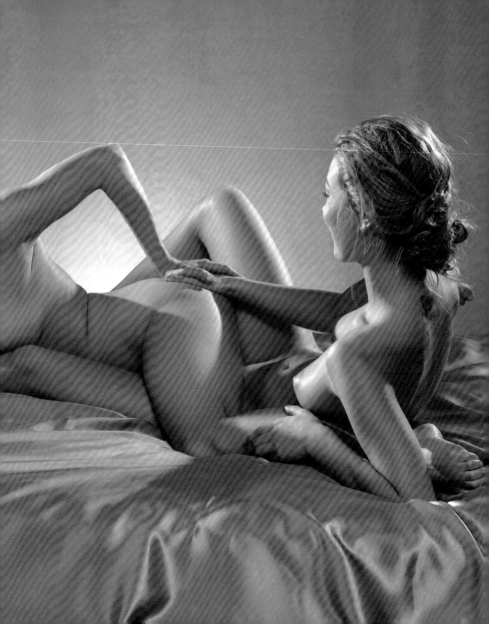

Reverse Scissors

Both partners are lying on their sides, with their heads on opposite ends of the bed. Their bodies are facing opposite directions. Their legs have slid open to allow their vulvas to touch, providing good frictional stimulation. If it's more comfortable, one partner can lie more on her stomach than her side.

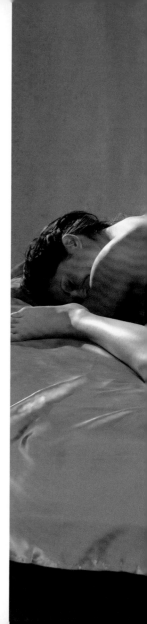

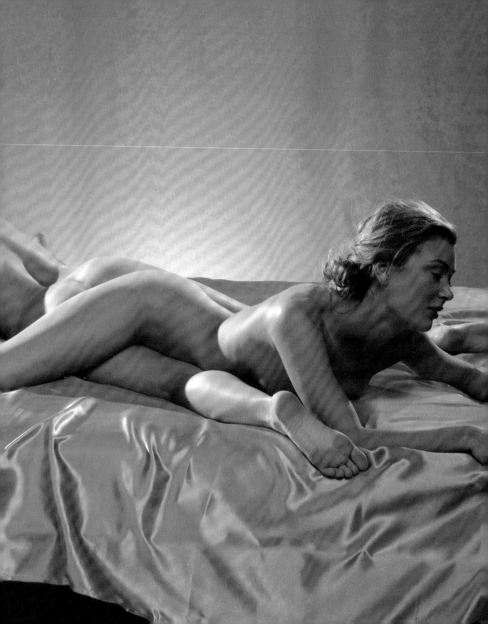

Sophisticated Scissors

Similar to the Reverse Scissors position, this fabulous-friction focused move has one of the partners sitting up in bed, resting her weight on her arm. This allows her both more control and more power as the two rub against each other's bodies... plus she gets a front row seat to watch her lover hit her climax. If they'd like, they can take turns sitting up to decide what feels best for the two of them, and to share the best view in the house!

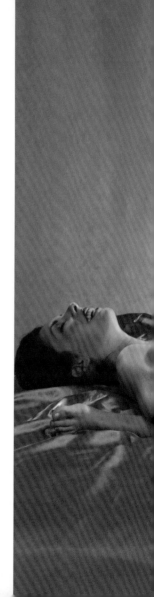

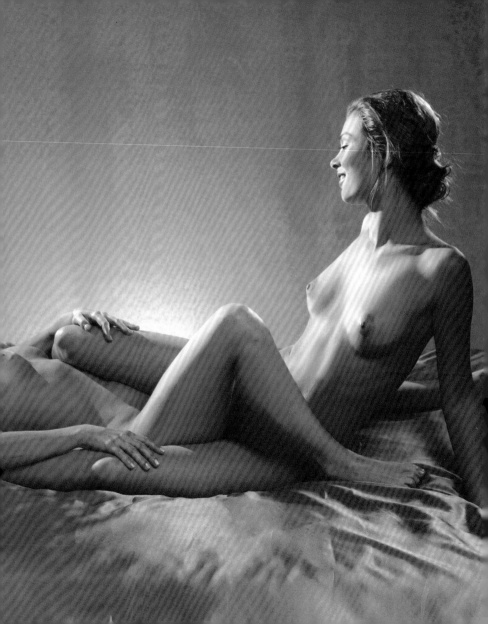

This Is the Way the Ladies Ride

One woman is sitting on a chair, with her legs at a right angle to the floor, slightly spread apart at the feet. The other woman is straddling one of the sitting partner's legs while she's facing her partner. Wrapping her arms around the woman in the chair, the riding partner is rubbing her vulva against the leg she's on. They can also play with each other's nipples, kiss, and so on while in this position.

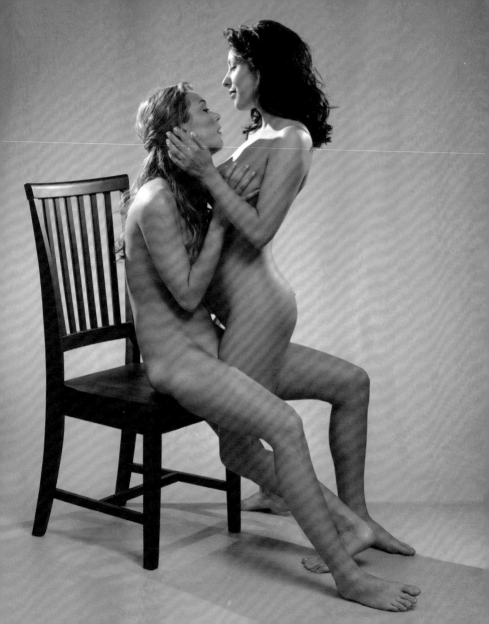

Bridge to Ecstasy

With one woman sitting on the bed with her legs out in a V (or one leg can be bent at the knee), her partner is able to straddle the outstretched leg and rub herself along it at the speed and pace that feels best to her. This position allows for eye contact, kissing, and real intimacy, while letting the woman straddling the leg have complete control over her own stimulation.

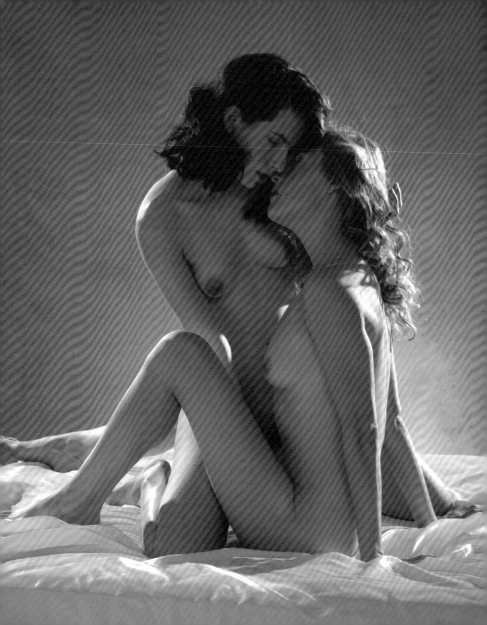

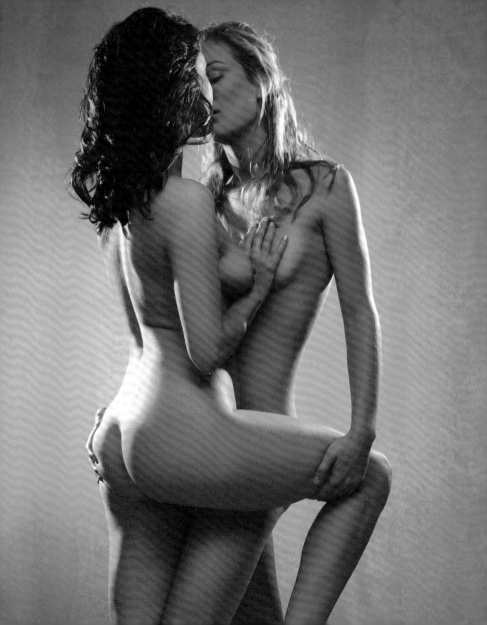

Lean on Me

Both partners are standing and facing each other, with one placing her leg between her partner's legs. She then lifts up and holds one of her partner's legs at a right angle by her hip, allowing for deeper access and more friction to be achieved. Either partner can move to create scintillating stimulation, or they can rock back and forth together to really rock her world!

Fits Like a Glove

The partners are lying in the traditional spooning position, on their sides, facing the same direction. The woman in back has her arm wrapped around the waist of the woman in front. They can grind against each other, and the woman in the front can stimulate herself with her fingers or a toy. The women can also lift their legs over each other to provide more surface area to rub against.

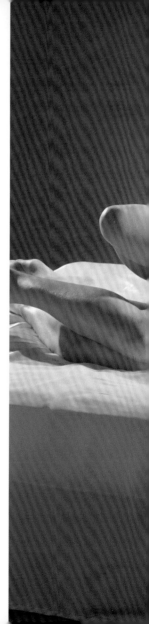

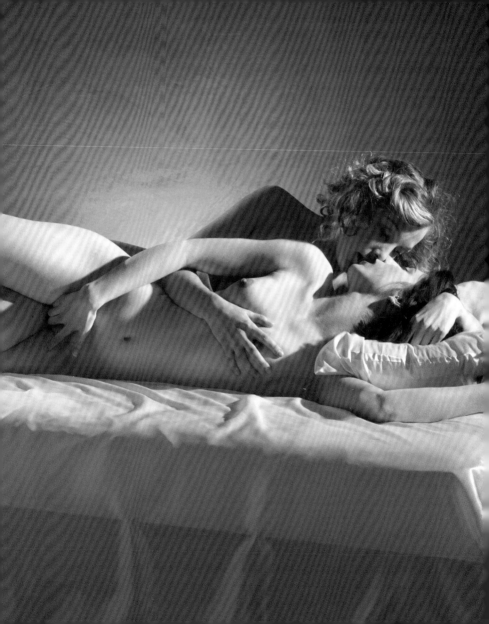

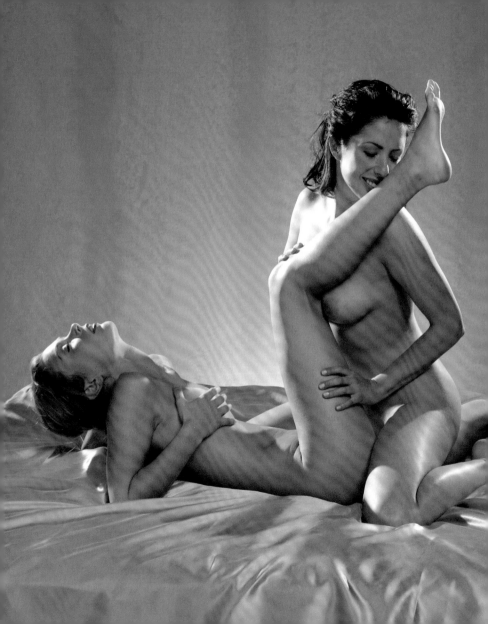

Work It On Up

One woman is lying on her back on the bed, propped up on her elbows so she can see her partner. One leg is flat on the bed, the other is up in the air and can be resting on her partner if comfortable. Her partner is straddling her just below the open leg, facing her, so that her vulva can rub up against the first partner's thigh/back of the leg. The straddling partner can be kneeling or even squatting, whichever feels better for her, and she's supporting her partner's leg in the air. The woman lying on her back can reach down and stimulate her partner's vulva as well.

Deep Lotus

A position that allows for both partners to rub against each other, with one woman on her back, her legs open, spread, and bent at the knees. Her partner kneels in between these spread legs with her knees slightly apart, pressing up into her. She can lean forward to kiss, or use her arms to change the angle and therefore the sensations between them. Requires some degree of flexibility.

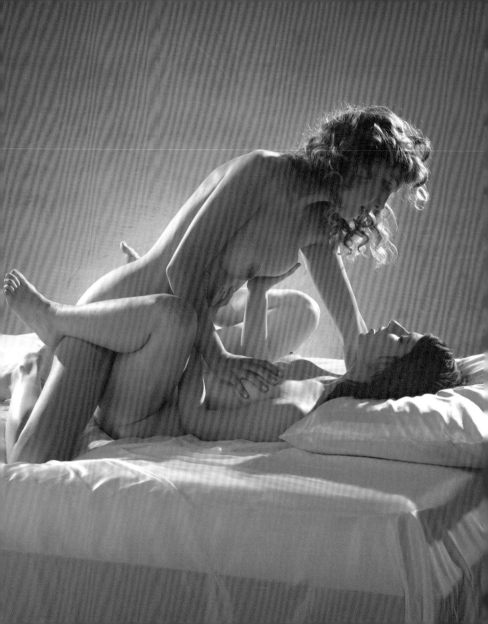

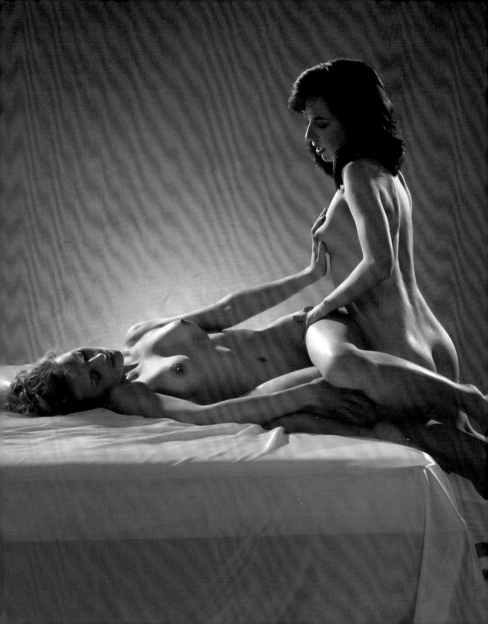

Side Saddle

One partner is lying near the edge of the bed on her side, with her knees bent and relaxed. Her partner comes up, standing on one leg, and places her other leg between the knees of the partner who is on her side on the bed, so that both of them are providing friction up against each other. Use a pillow or two under the hips of the partner on the bed to change up the angle for different sensations.

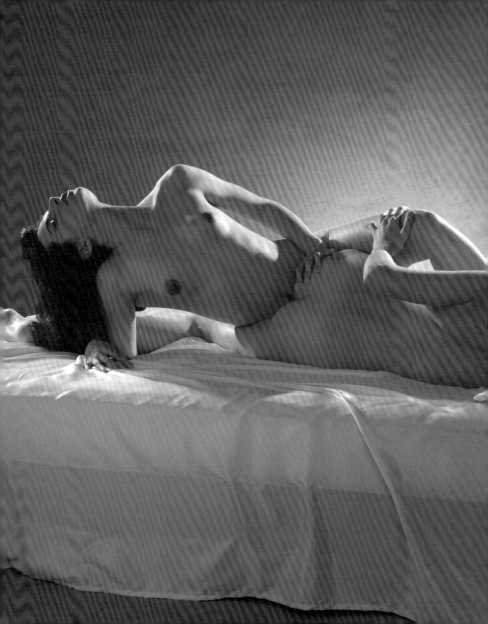

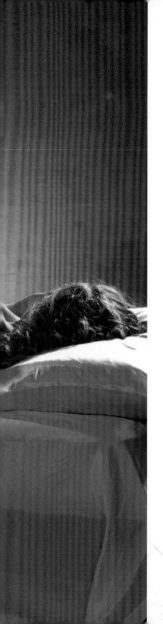

Intimately Entwined

Both partners are lying in bed on their sides, facing each other. One woman places her leg over the other woman's hip and slides her other leg between her partner's leg. They can now rub their vulvas on each other's legs. This is a great position for intimacy: they can look at each other, kiss, play with each other's nipples, and so on, all while enjoying rubbing up on each other.

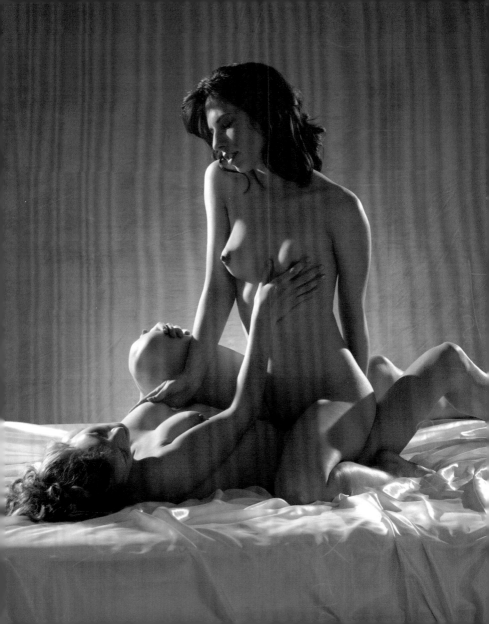

The Raunchy Rodeo

Somewhat emulating the more traditional "cowgirl" position, one woman is lying on her back on the bed while the other has straddled her waist. She can then either kneel or squat and move up and down or side to side to provide frictional pleasure for them both. This position allows for kissing, eye contact, breast stimulation, and all sorts of additional intimacy.

Spooning Cowgirl

One woman is sitting on a chair with her legs at a right angle to the floor, feet slightly spread apart. The other woman is straddling one of her legs, with her back to her partner, in almost a reverse cowgirl style. The woman sitting in the chair has wrapped her arms around the woman riding her (and can choose to play with her riding partner's nipples), as the riding woman is rubbing her vulva against the leg she's on.

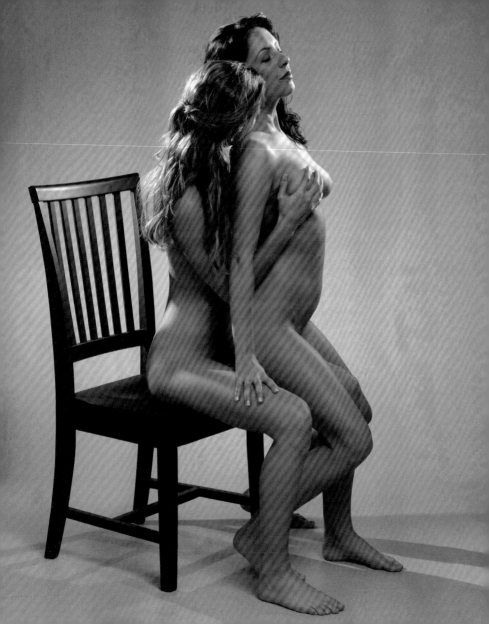

Sliding into Home

Another position that allows the top partner complete control, this position has one woman lying on her back with one leg straight and the other bent at the knee, and a pillow propped up under her head. The other woman lies on her, straddling her bent leg with her vulva, rubbing up against the leg, and across the woman on the bed's body. It gives the woman on top control over the sensations she is getting, but allows them both to connect more through constant touch.

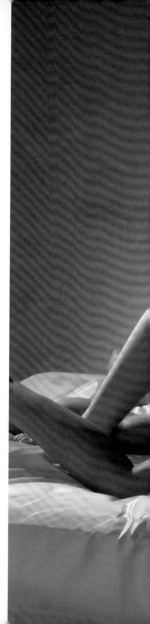

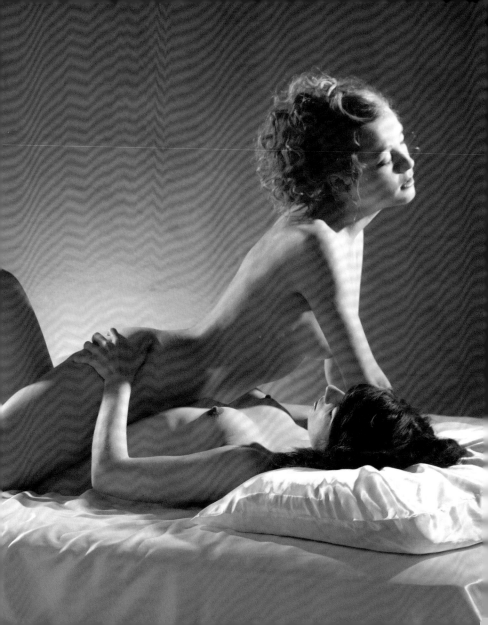

Absolute X-tasy

This position may be a little more challenging, but can certainly be worth it for those who crave simultaneous and direct stimulation. One woman is lying on the bed on her back, supporting herself in almost a bridge with one knee bent. The other is standing, sliding between her partner's legs, holding up one of her partner's knees next to her body while using her non-standing leg to bend and straighten in order to control the pace. Their legs together form an X.

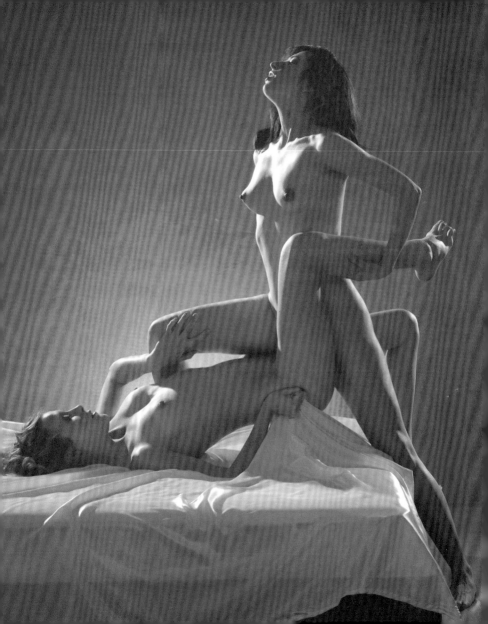

Stacked Spoons

One woman is lying on the bed on her stomach, with her head turned to the side (it can be resting on a pillow, or she can even put a pillow below her chest if that's more comfortable). Her partner is lying almost on top of her, but a bit more to the side, supporting herself slightly with her arms and sliding her vulva against the first woman's back for stimulation. This can be a relaxing, very laid-back position, great for warm-up or cool down.

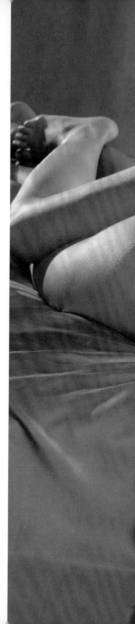

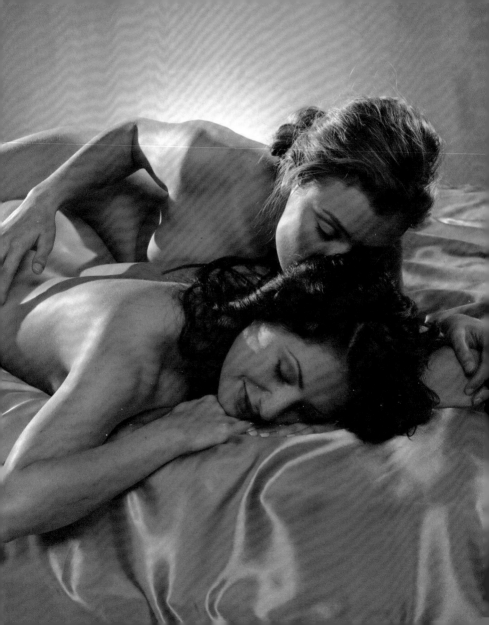

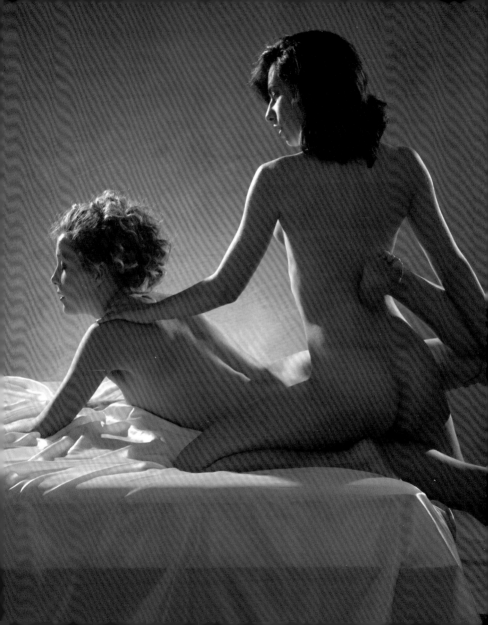

Erotic Arabesque

For partners who have a little bit of extra flexibility available to them, this position really stretches your limits. One partner is lying on the bed, semi-supporting herself with one leg hanging down. Her other leg is bent and pulled back by her partner who is half kneeling on the bed while straddling her other leg. This position really opens up the first woman's vulva, allowing for dual stimulation, and is satisfying everyone involved.

The Sensual Slide

With one partner lying on the bed, her knees bent and spread, the other partner straddles one of those bent legs, sliding her vulva up and down the leg to provide herself with pleasurable stimulation. The partner lying on the bed gets an excellent view of her lover's back as she faces away from her, while the straddling partner pleasures herself on the first partner's leg, and can reach down to stimulate herself by hand (or with a toy!) if she so chooses.

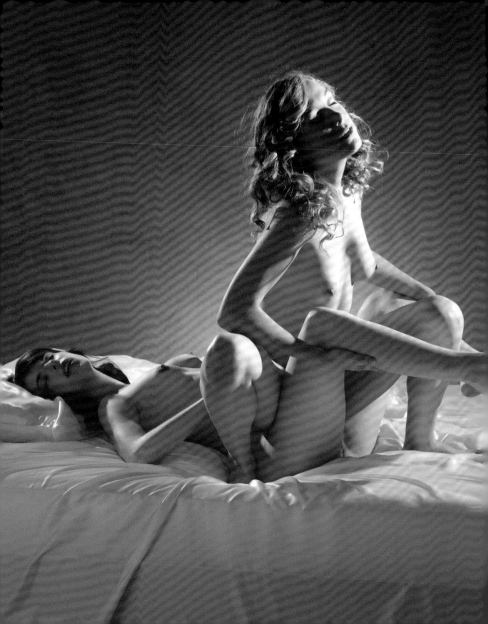

Riding High

Both partners are facing each other, lying on the bed, one lying on top of the other, with their legs essentially intertwined. The woman on top is straddling one of her partner's legs, pushing her body against the leg to stimulate her vulva, while her partner can choose to wrap her leg around for a different sensation. Very intimate, the partner on top is in control of her sensations, but they can maintain eye contact, kiss, and play with one another throughout.

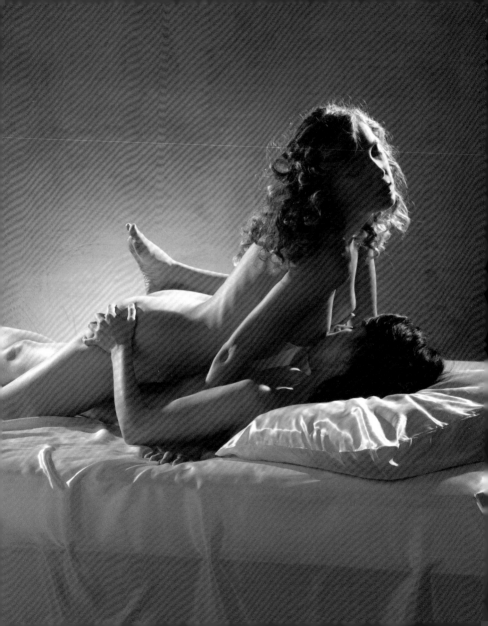

ORAL PASSION

Ah, cunnilingus. Dining at the Y. Licking alotta puss. Eating her out. Whatever you want to call it, oral sex on female bodies can be incredibly exciting and titillating. Regardless of whether you choose to use oral sex as foreplay, the main course, or a delicious helping of dessert, many folks enjoy both giving and receiving the art of cunnilingus.

If either of you are concerned about smell or taste, here are a few tips:

First, the shower is your friend. It doesn't matter how you actually smell or taste (which is probably pretty freaking awesome) if you're going to fret about it during sex. Cut these worries off at the pass by showering together first. This way, you both know that both of you are squeaky clean, it gives you some more exciting foreplay options like soaping each other up and rubbing each other down, and it can help both of you relax before the sexual exploration starts.

Think about what you eat. While there's no miracle diet for having a delicious vulva, some foods can make you taste more bitter and others leave you tasting sweeter. Fruits like pineapple, orange, and lemon, can give you that lighter flavor, while heavier or creamy foods (cream sauces, broccoli, asparagus) might give you a hint of a bitter taste. Garlic is on the fence; if you eat enough of it, your vulva may taste like it, so that really depends on whether your partner enjoys garlic or might be turned off.

Finally, keep in mind that you're supposed to taste like you. All of us have our own individual flavor and scent. You're not supposed to smell like a rose or taste like a mint julep; this is sex, not perfume. Many folks love the way their partner naturally smells and tastes, so if you're concerned, ask before you start spritzing on weird sprays that mess with your pH and can leave you with a bacterial infection.

If you want safer oral sex, you can use a dam, or make your own! What's a dam? It's a very thin sheet of latex (similar in feeling to a condom) that's rectangular. You lube up the area to be licked, then place the dam on top of it, and go at it! The problem with dams is that they tend to be hard to find, expensive, and not great for those with latex sensitivities.

It's time to MacGyver your safer sex supplies! Take an unrolled condom and cut it in half, from tip to the base (lengthwise). Voilà—you have a mini dam, and you can even use flavored condoms, lubricated or not, or nonlatex condoms.

Another great trick is to take a glove (latex, nitrile, or vinyl), cut off the four finger spaces and up the NON-thumb side. Open it, and now you have a dam with a little finger hole for you to stimulate inside as well.

Ta-da! Gloves are cheap en masse, and you can find them at grocery stores, drugstores, or even beauty supply shops.

Another easy-to-make alternative is to use plastic wrap from the kitchen. Most people already have this on hand, it comes in a variety of pretty colors, and you can actually see what's beneath the wrap and enjoy what you're licking. All plastic wrap is latex-free, so it's preferable for use, regardless of whether you or your partner has a latex allergy.

Don't forget that good cunnilingus takes time. I'm not saying that you need to put aside two hours for muff diving (unless it really turns both you and your partner on that much; if so, feel free to dedicate your whole day!), but you do need to remember that it'll likely take more than a minute, or even five, to get things going. There's no magic recipe for giving good head, but communication and enthusiasm are the two sure bets you have for making it as good as it can possibly be. Ask for feedback (and make sure to give it, if you're the receiver!), and show your partner exactly how much you want to be there, whether you're the one licking or the one lying back and enjoying it. Keep in mind that using pillows can help make both partners significantly more comfortable, and that different people enjoy their oral stimulation in different positions. Mix things up, and you're sure to have a fabulous time.

Intimate Inversion

The woman receiving the oral sex is lying on the bed, mostly on her back, with her weight resting on her shoulders, neck, and head, supported by her arms. Her hips are in the air, with her feet resting over her partner's shoulders, and can be crossed at the ankles. Her partner then is resting on her knees, her hands and arms supporting the receiving partner's butt and back, allowing her comfortable face-level access to all of the areas to be licked, nibbled, and sucked. Consider adding pillows to make things more comfortable for either partner.

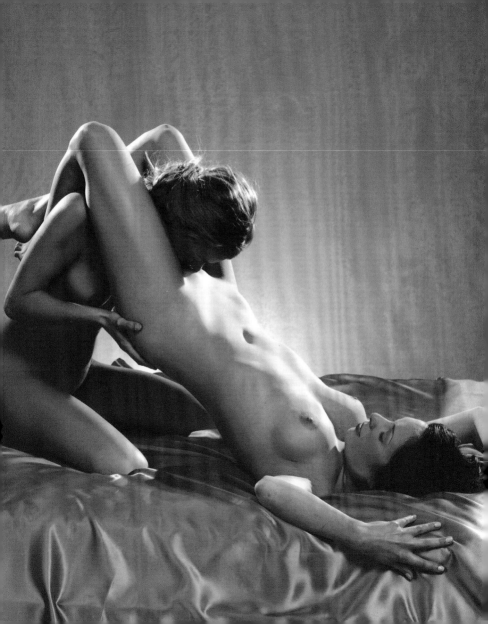

The Tantalizing Tangle

A position that allows both partners to delight each other with oral ministrations simultaneously, it is similar to a 69 but the pillow below the bottom partner's head allows her much better access to her partner's vulva (try two or even three pillows to find out what fits best). This position is a great way for both women to give and receive pleasure at the same time while allowing for the comfort of all involved.

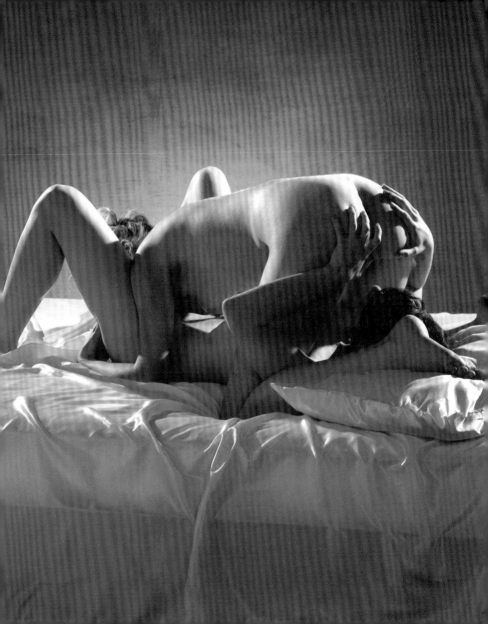

Temple of the Goddess

One partner is lying on the bed on her back, with her knees tucked towards her chest, but open slightly, using her hands to hold her knees in place. Her partner is also on the bed, kneeling between her legs, providing her with tantalizing oral pleasure. This position is a great one not only because of the access provided and the ability of the receiver to rock side to side slightly to best get her ideal stimulation, but also in playing with power, and having the giver provide oral sex in a somewhat submissive position.

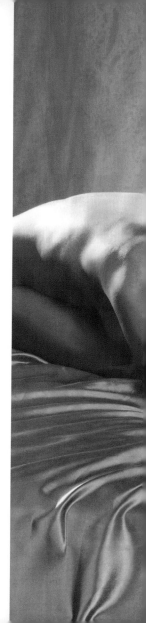

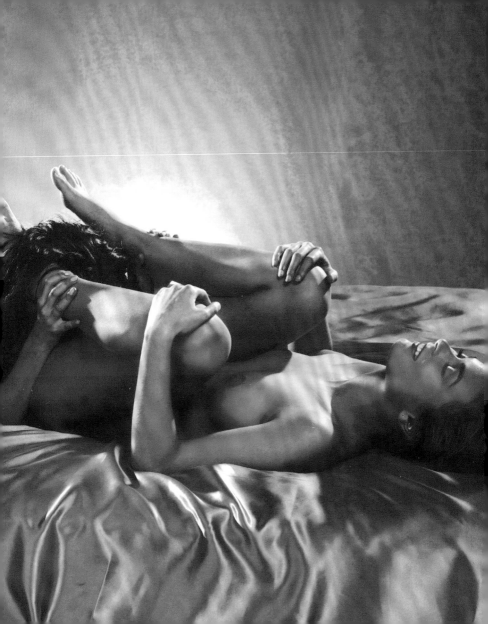

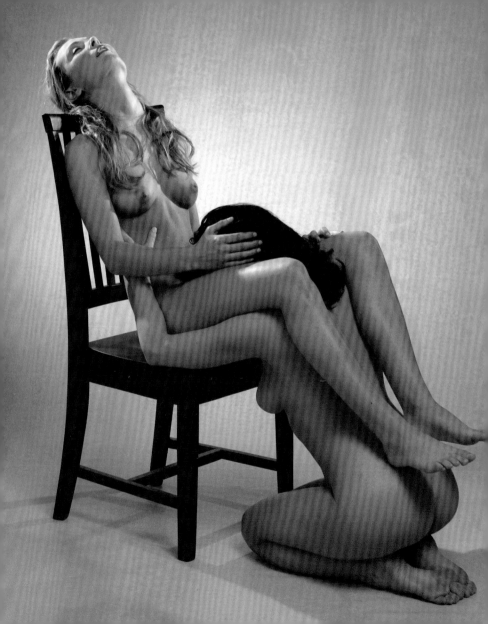

Worshipping Venus

The partner receiving the oral pleasure is sitting in a chair (find one with four legs; this is not a great position for a rocking or spinning chair!), leaning back slightly. Her partner is kneeling on the ground in front of her, facing the chair, with the sitting partner's legs over the kneeling partner's back. This gives both partners access to great angles that can really elevate pleasure, and it can be very comfortable for the receiver. Add a pillow under the giver's knees if it gets to be less than comfy.

Easy as Pie

The woman receiving oral sex is lying on her back on the bed with her legs open. Her legs can either be flat or bent at the knee with her feet on the bed, in case she'd like to move her hips around. Her partner lies between her legs, with her face between them and her arms around the legs to pull her closer if she'd like. The woman on her back can reach forward and put her hands in her partner's hair, or this could be a fun position to use for having her wrists restrained.

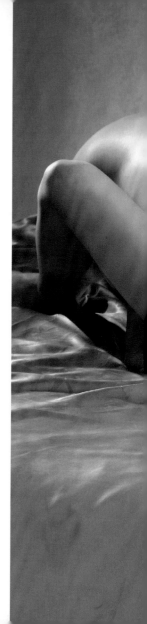

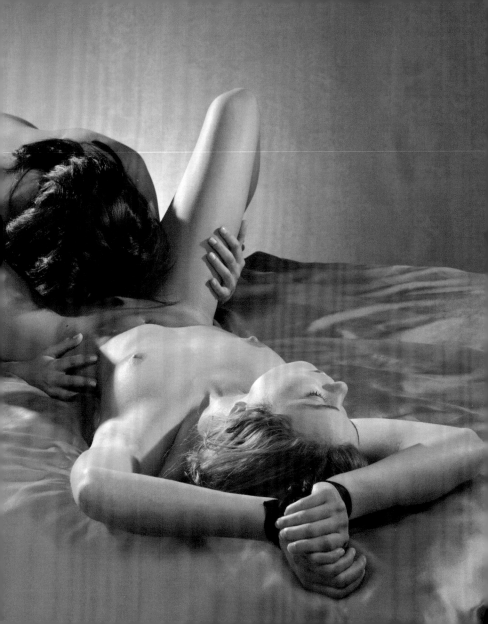

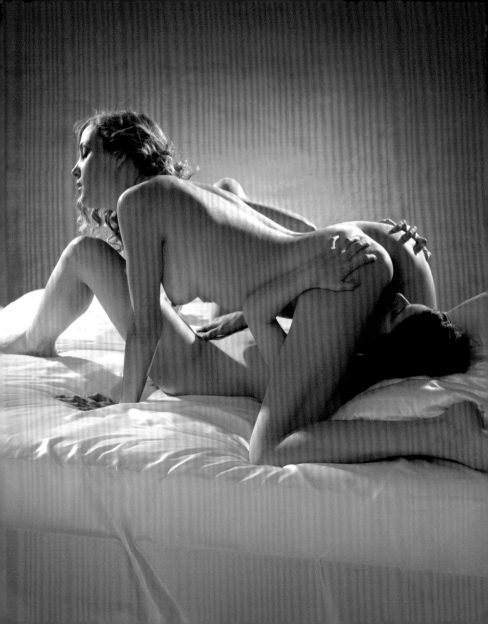

Palatable Pleasure

Similar to the beginnings of a 69 position, in this position the partner on top is supporting herself with one hand while using her free hand to stimulate the partner who is on the bed's vulva. The partner on the bed has both hands as well as her mouth free to pleasure her lover. This is a great position to add in a sex toy or two in addition to your oral skills, and also for some power play, with the partner on top being in a little more of a dominant role. Add a pillow under the bottom partner's head and/or hips to change up the angles!

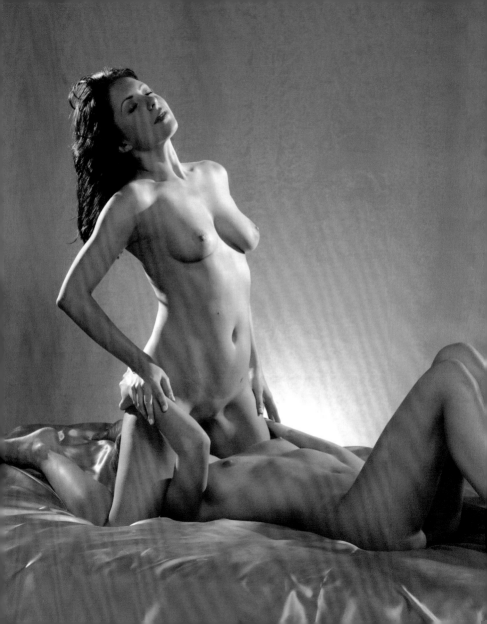

Classy Chassis

One woman is on the bed on her knees, her knees slightly spread, straddling her partner's face. Her partner is lying on the bed on her back with her legs out in front, licking upward (positioned like a car mechanic). The licker can place a pillow under her head to provide a better angle, and the receiver can lean forward more onto the bed if that's more comfortable for her. As shown, this is a good position to add some bondage if you so choose!

Open Wide

One woman is on her back on the bed, her legs opened wide. She has her arms holding her ankles to support keeping them up and open. Her partner is lying on her stomach between her partner's legs, with both arms wrapped around her legs from underneath to pull her closer to her face. Placing a pillow under the receiver's hips can provide a different angle that might work better for some folks.

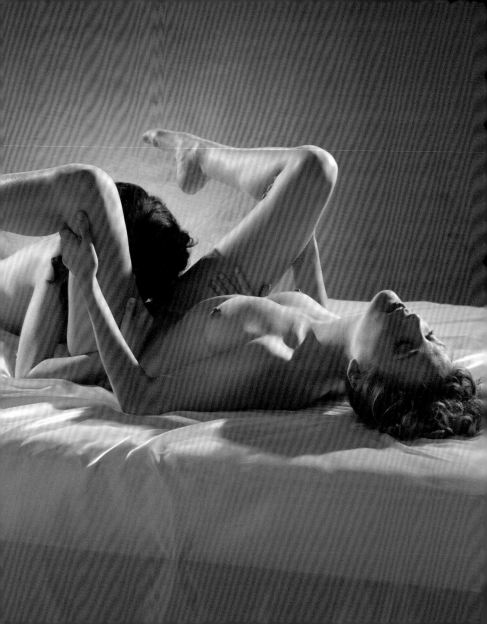

Blinded by Delight

The receiving partner is lying on her back on the bed, legs spread, wearing a blindfold. Her partner is lying between her legs, her head positioned for optimal licking pleasure. The woman on her back can wrap her legs around her partner, and the licker can reach up to stimulate the breasts or hold her partner's hands. Losing one sense, like sight, can heighten all the other senses and significantly increase pleasure.

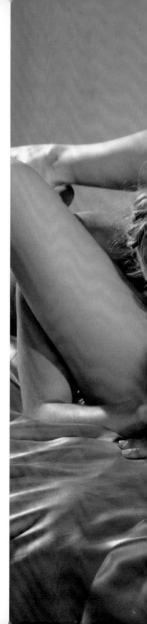

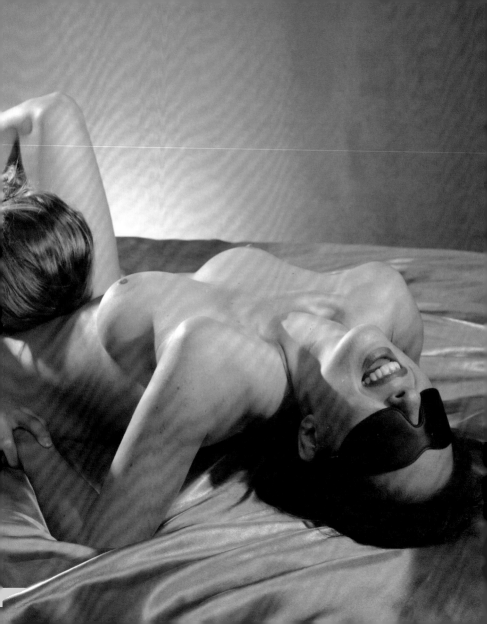

The Salacious Straddle

With one woman lying flat on the bed, the other woman kneels facing the first woman's feet, putting one of her knees on each side of the first partner's head. During the course of receiving oral stimulation, she can either stay kneeling with her body straight up, or can lean forward and support herself with her arms, depending on which angle feels better to her. The partner on the bed can reach up to stimulate the riding partner's breasts, or she can reach down and play with herself while giving pleasure.

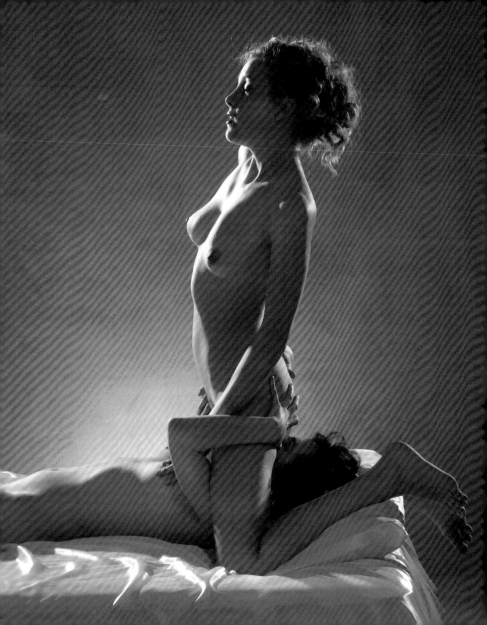

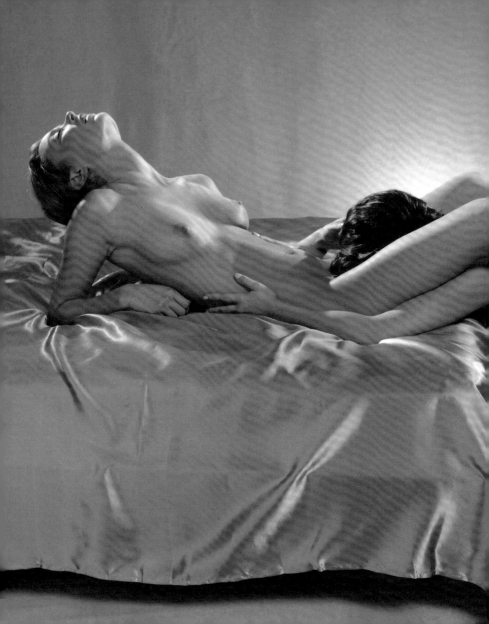

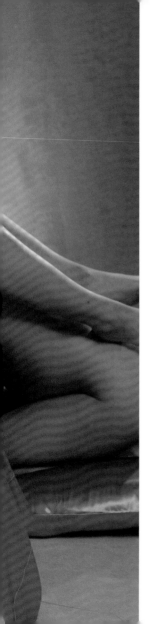

Kneeling Worship

One woman is on the floor at the edge of the bed, kneeling, facing the bed. The other woman is on the edge of the bed, sitting up straight, resting her open legs on her partner's shoulders, her partner's head in front of her vulva. One or both of her hands can be wrapped in her partner's hair or holding her partner's head, or she can use one or both hands to support her body on the bed. Having her feet on her partner's shoulders allows for a better view, and, of course, more intimate access to her vulva.

Riding into the Night

One woman is lying on her back on the bed. The other woman is facing the wall, with her knees on either side of her partner's head as she's straddling her face. She can have one or both hands on the wall, supporting her. The woman on the bed can help steady the rider by placing her hands on her hips and also pull her closer or push her away as needed.

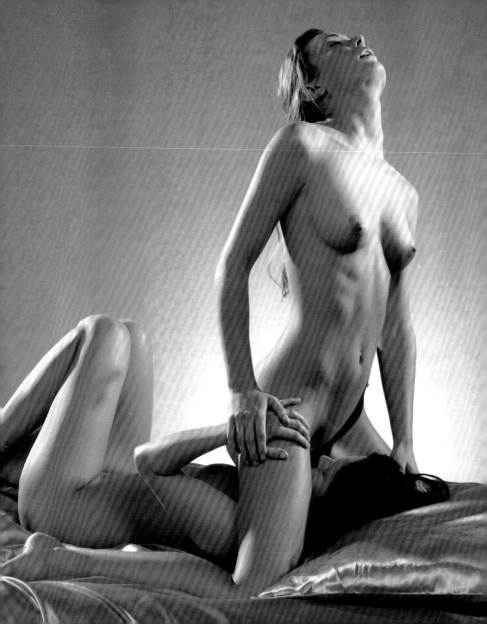

Have a Leg Up

The receiving woman stands at the edge of the bed, facing the bed. She's standing on one leg and the other leg is placed on the bed with a bent knee. Her partner can be sitting on the floor or a chair (depending on the bed's height), licking her and helping the standing woman to keep her balance. They can both touch each other for additional sensations and support, and the giver can use a vibrator to keep her partner stimulated while she's providing oral sex, if she so desires.

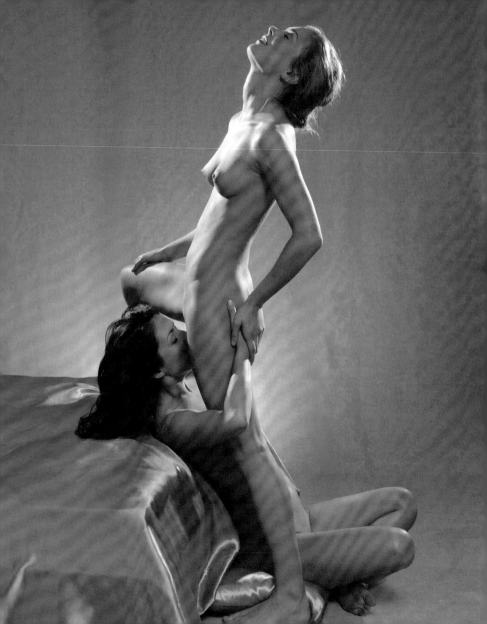

Orgasmic Earmuffs

One woman is lying on her side. Her bottom leg is straight with her top leg bent up to make a triangle. She has placed her foot on her knee, and she's supporting herself slightly on a bent arm, looking down. Her partner is lying on her side, her head in the vulva area, resting her head on the first woman's thigh, body facing toward her head. This might look like a T from above. The thigh helps provide a place for the licker to rest her head during the oral action.

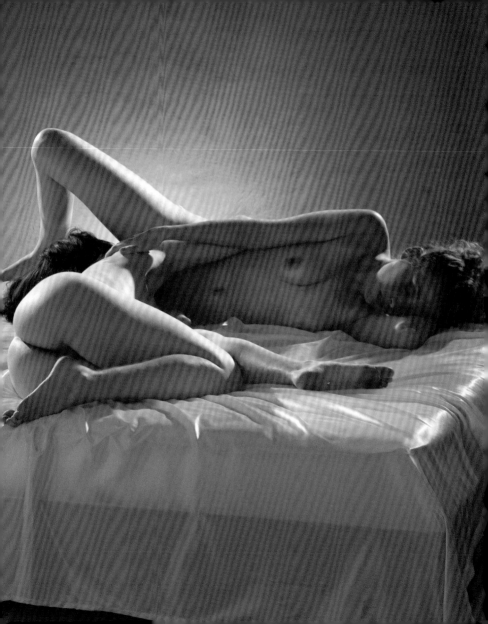

Sexy Somersault

In some ways like the traditional 69 position, this one really kicks it up a notch. Designed for those with a little extra flexibility, one partner is on the bed on her back, bent in half while holding her ankles with her hand. The other partner is kneeling on either side of her head, allowing access to her vulva while also leaning forward to give her lover oral pleasure. If needed, pillows can be used to help prop one or the other woman in place and make things more comfortable.

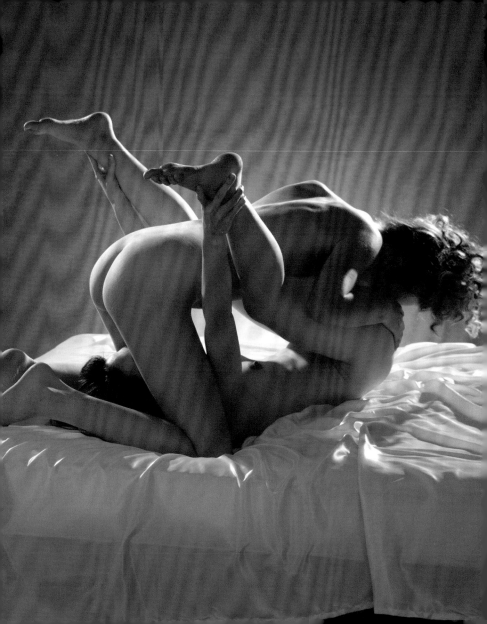

Up the Wall

One woman is standing with her back against the wall. Her legs are spread, and her arms are reaching along her sides to balance her. The other woman is sitting cross-legged between the receiver's legs, facing the wall. She has placed both hands on the receiver's hips, pulling her vulva close to her face for optimal licking. The sitting woman may choose to place a pillow or other item under her for added comfort.

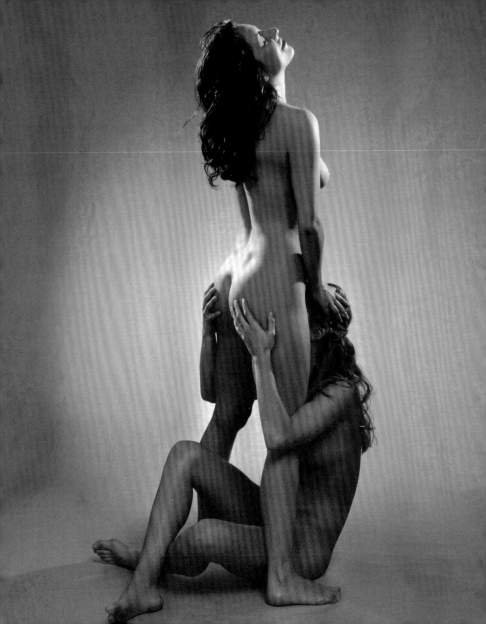

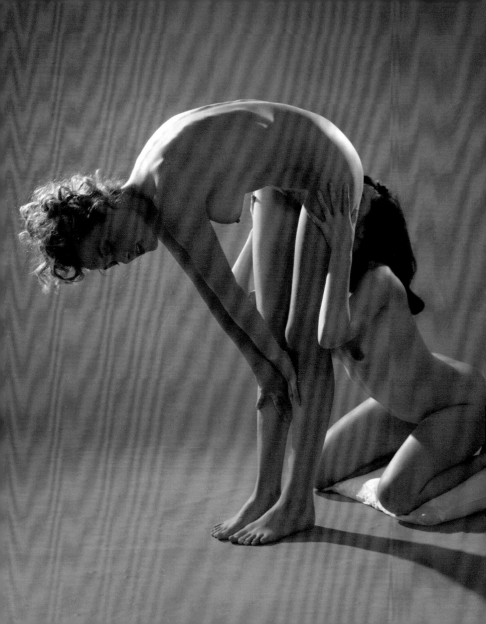

Forward Fold

The woman receiving oral sex is bent over at the waist, her hands on her ankles and her legs shoulder-width apart. Her partner is on her knees behind the standing woman, holding the standing woman's hips with her hands, and has her face near her vulva from the rear. This can also be a great position for analingus. The kneeling partner may want to place a pillow under her knees if it's more comfortable.

Flying First Class

One of the women is lying on her back, with her head at the end of the bed. The other woman is either kneeling over or even straddling her face, allowing her feet to hang off the side of the bed (with lower beds, they can be placed over the edge of the bed and then flat on the floor for additional leverage). This allows for increased access to the vulva, and also power play as the woman on top controls access and even breath play with the woman below.

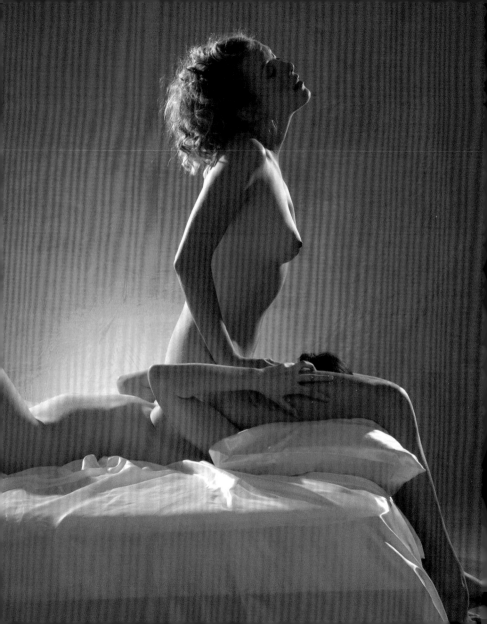

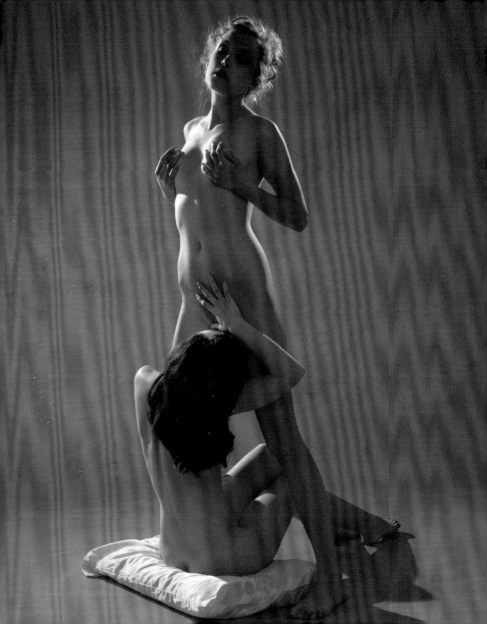

Leg Over Easy

One woman is sitting on the ground, cross-legged, with her back straight. The other woman is standing, facing her partner, with one leg straddled over her partner's back, allowing the sitting partner access to her vulva. The standing woman's hands can be bracing herself on the wall, placed on her partner's shoulders, or holding onto her partner's head. The sitting partner can help steady the standing one and also use her hands to move the standing woman's vulva to the best area for licking.

Traditional 69

One woman is lying on her back on the bed, with her head resting on some pillows. The other woman has her legs or knees spread on either side of the first woman's shoulders, facing her partner's body, with her head near her partner's vulva. Both women have access to each other's vulvas and can be licking, sucking, and stimulating each other at the same time.

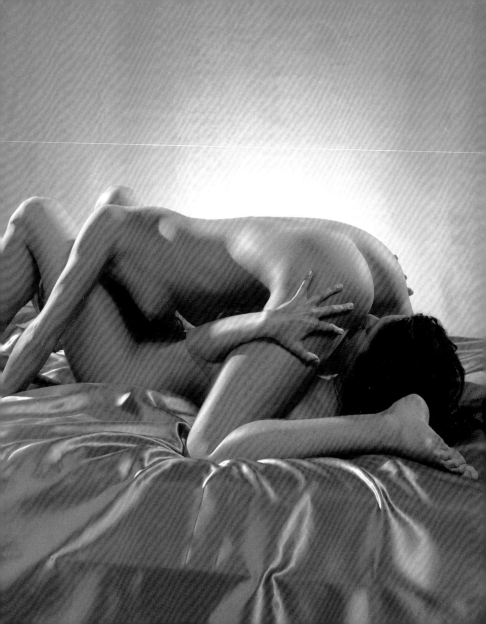

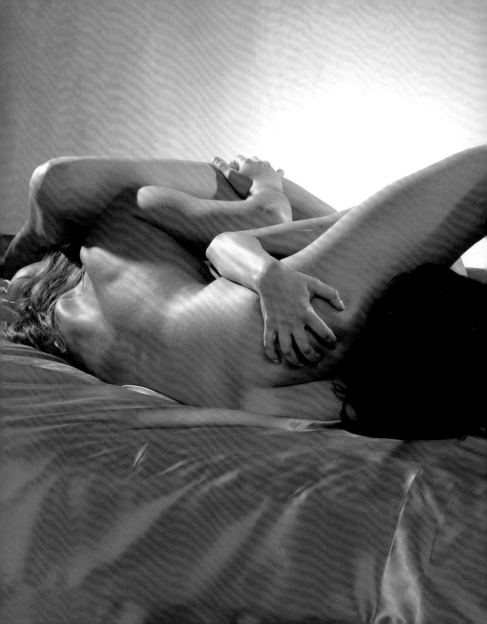

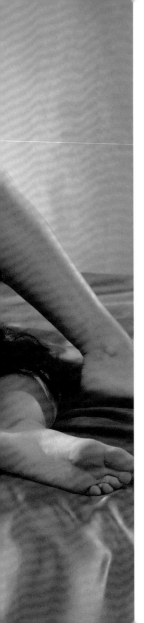

Sliding Spoons

One woman is on her side with her bottom leg straight out, and her top leg bent with her foot on her knee or the bed. Her partner is also lying on her side, facing the first woman, but with her head between her legs. This places her own legs near the first woman's face for possible 69 action. They can both use pillows to support their heads and get their necks at the right angles for licking each other.

Sweet Handiwork

The licker is lying on the bed, on her back, with her head resting on some pillows. The other woman has her legs (mostly knees) spread on either side of her partner's shoulders as she faces her body. She's supporting herself with one arm and using the other to manually stimulate her partner, while the woman lying down is providing oral and potentially manual stimulation to the kneeling partner.

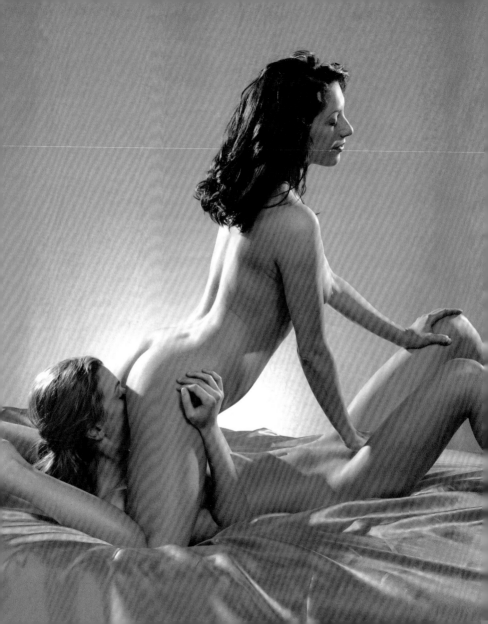

ANAL AFFECTIONS

Here's the lowdown about anal: like all sexual activities, some people love it, some people hate it, and some people are on the fence. While bodies that are assigned female at birth don't have prostates, people of all sexes and genders can enjoy anal sex, if that's a sensation they enjoy. On the other hand, there are some people (including those with prostates) for whom anal sex is blasé, or even triggering, and for those folks, it's probably a good idea to let this idea go and move on to the next exciting sexual adventure.

Let's say that you and your partner have decided you're both excited about trying out anal stimulation. Excellent: way to be using some fabulous two-way communication. Start slow. Anal sex is definitely a journey, and not a "wham, bam, thank you, ma'am" kind of goal. If the person receiving the anal action is new to backdoor play, then it's more important that you go super slow and get good feedback. If you (or they) have never had anything in your bottom, don't decide that a big, thick dildo is the best way to start things. Rather, a lubed-up pinky finger or some silicone butt beads are a better way to begin.

Make sure you choose toys that you can sterilize, which means they're 100 percent silicone, glass, metal, or ceramic. Using toys like this, with lots of lube, is a great way to warm up the butt, either by yourself prior to playtime or with a partner.

It's important to remember lubrication during any type of anal penetration. The anus has no natural lubrication, so not lubing up before playing with it can lead to microtears and cuts. If you're just using your fingers (or non-silicone toys), you can choose between silicone- and water-based lube, versus just water-based lube if silicone toys are in play.

The anus, unlike the vagina, has no end to it. This means that anything you put in the anus needs to have a flanged base, meaning the base is wider than the rest of the toy. All dildos designed for harnesses have a flanged base. Butt plugs do as well (they are meant to go in and stay in, rather than go in and out). Be wary of butt beads that are connected by string: they can break. If something DOES get lost in your bottom, you have a couple of hours to try and relax, and then try to get it out. After that, head to the ER.

Anal sex, of any kind, is not supposed to hurt. If it hurts, something's wrong, and that's your body's way of telling you to slow down, back off, and try something different. This is why you should stay away from numbing gels; if your body can't tell you something's wrong, you'll keep going, and you can cause anal tears or other issues without even feeling it. Instead, add more lube, take some deep breaths, offer feedback on what feels good, what doesn't feel good, and what you need, and back off for a while if things keep hurting. For some women, enjoying other types of stimulation, and even orgasms, before anal play can make the anal exploration even more enjoyable. Just remember: there's no right way to have anal sex, but if it hurts, there's definitely a wrong way.

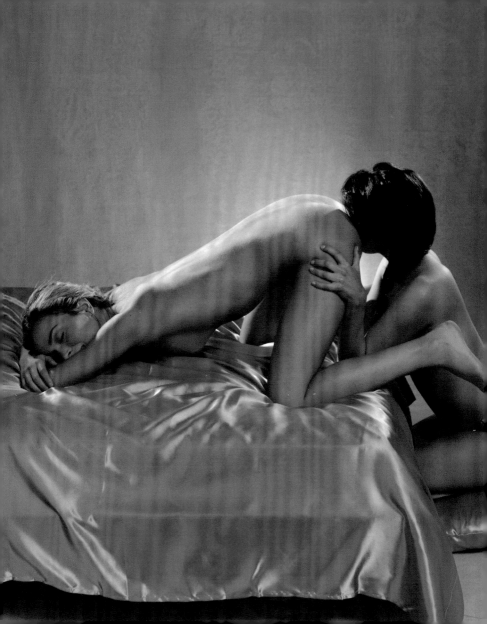

Kissing the Rosebud

One woman is kneeling doggy-style on the edge of the bed, leaning either on her hands or on her elbows. Her partner is kneeling on the floor behind her, holding her hips, and using her mouth and tongue to stimulate the anus. She can also reach up and play with the receiver's breasts and nipples if she'd like. The woman on the floor can use a pillow under her knees, if she so desires, for additional comfort.

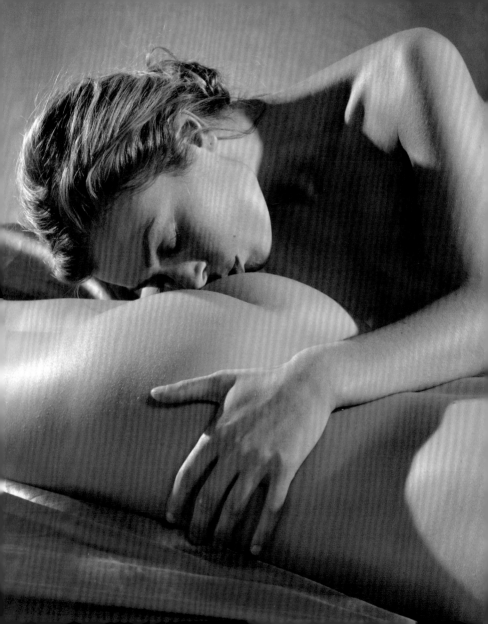

Loving Licks

One woman is lying on her stomach on the bed, using pillows under her head, chest, and hips to get as comfortable as possible. Her partner is sitting next to her on the bed, leaning forward to kiss her butt cheeks before gently spreading them to provide analingus, and maybe a finger or two of penetration. The woman on her stomach can reach below her body with fingers or a vibrator to give herself additional clitoral stimulation during playtime.

Back It On Up

The woman receiving the anal penetration is on her knees on the bed in a doggy-style position, either propping herself up on her hands or elbows, whichever is more comfortable. Her partner is on her knees behind her, wearing a strap-on, penetrating her anally. This is a great position for anal newbies, as the person getting penetrated can slowly back up onto the dildo to receive the depth of penetration that's comfortable for her, and she can also use her hands and elbows to change the angle of her body for more pleasure. The person doing the penetration can reach around and stimulate her partner's clitoris with fingers or a vibrator, or can lean forward to pull her hair or play with her breasts.

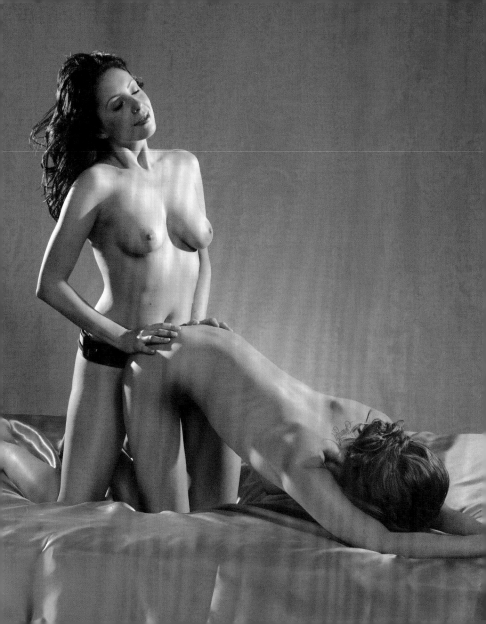

Backdoor Rodeo

One woman is lying on the bed on her back, wearing a harness. She can put a pillow under her head if she'd like more comfort and a better viewing angle. The other woman straddles her partner, facing away from her, and while either kneeling or squatting, lowers herself onto the dildo anally. She can choose the speed, depth, and angle of penetration by lowering faster or slower, leaning forward or backward, and pushing herself up more. The partner on the bed gets quite a good show!

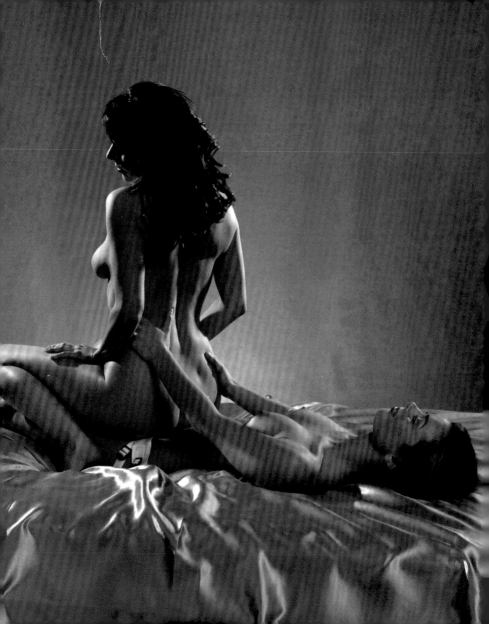

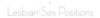

The Right Angle

The woman receiving the anal penetration is on her knees on the bed, supporting herself on her forearms or hands as she leans forward to form a triangle with her body and the bed. Her partner is behind her, wearing a strap-on. She's on her knees, penetrating her lover anally, with her hands on the receiver's hips, pulling her onto the strap-on. One or both women can place pillows beneath their knees for added comfort.

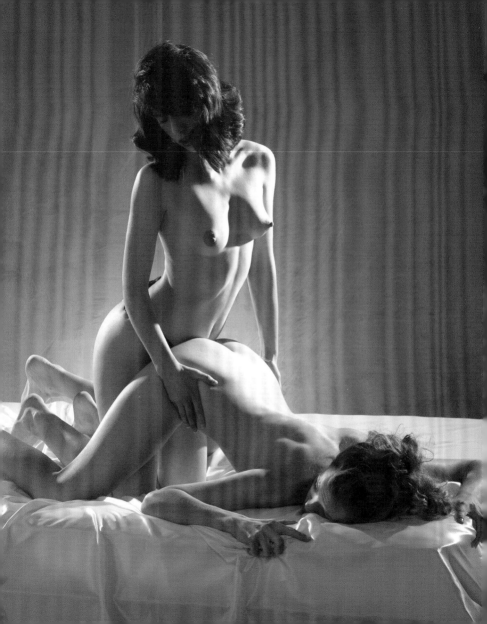

Stick 'Em Up!

One woman is standing, facing the wall. Her legs are spread, and her hands are flat on the wall above her head or resting on a chair in front of her for additional balance if she needs it. Her partner is on the floor, kneeling behind her (placing a pillow beneath her knees can make it more comfortable), supporting herself by placing her hands on the standing woman's hips. She's leaning forward so that her lips are buried between her standing partner's butt cheeks. For more access, the standing partner can move her feet wider apart or back away from the wall so that she can bend forward a bit more.

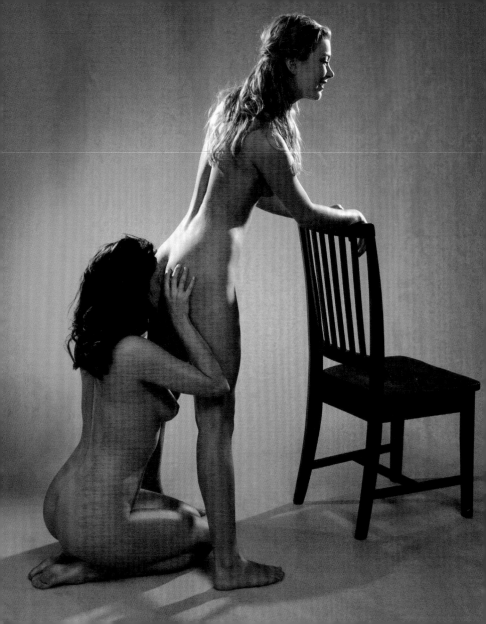

Face-Off

The partner wearing the harness and dildo is lying on her back on the bed, her head on a pillow, with her legs extended out in front of her. Her partner is straddling her in a cowgirl-like position, allowing herself to be anally penetrated. They can hold hands, play with each other's breasts, and even stimulate each other's vulvas with fingers or toys. The woman being penetrated can control the speed and depth of the thrusting, allowing her control over the movement.

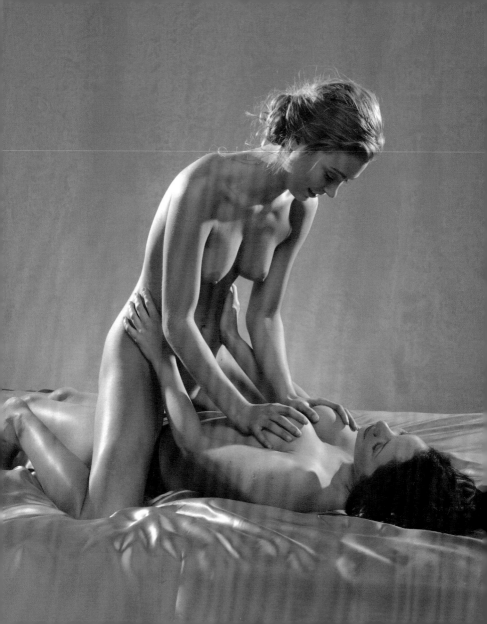

STRAP-ON PLAY

WHAT EXACTLY IS "A STRAP-ON"?

Harnesses come in various sizes, styles, and materials. There's no "right" harness, but there's one that's right for you. They're leather, pleather, vinyl, nylon webbing and faux velvet, just nylon webbing, swimsuitlike material, rope, rubber, and other options. Choose the material that works best for you. Some people have multiple harnesses of different materials, either for different partners or activities. Different harnesses fit different sizes; if you're curvier, make sure it adjusts to fit you. If you're slimmer, make sure you can get it tight.

A popular style is the thong-style/single strap, which goes around your hips and has just one strap threaded through your legs. Many women like this configuration because it offers some clitoral rubbing while you're wearing it. Some don't like this style because they either don't like the feeling or want more access to their own vulva during sex.

The other popular style is the jock-style/two strap, with two leg straps that fit firmly around your butt cheeks, like a stylized jockstrap. Some think this style is too sporty; others enjoy the support it provides, the adjustability, and the access provided to the wearer during sex.

While those harnesses are the easiest to find, there are other options out there should you wish to experiment. Options include thigh harnesses, palm harness, chest harnesses, boot harnesses, chin harnesses, forehead harnesses, and more. Truly, you can strap it on any which way you like.

The other piece: the dildo. While "dildo" is the technical term, people use a variety of words here: cock, dong, woo-woo, faux penis, and so on. Like every other type of sexual terminology, there's not a right or wrong word. Use whichever word (or words) make you and your partner hot.

Dildos come in a huge spectrum of sizes, shapes, colors, and designs. As long as it has a flat base that will allow you to use it in your harness, you can choose pretty much any dildo you want. When choosing one, make sure you take the person who will be penetrated into account; you might picture your strap-on cock being 12 inches and purple, while your partner might be wanting and needing something a bit more petite and with sparkles. Keep in mind that our eyes tend to be bigger than our vaginas; it's always easy to add more size, and it's much harder to take it away. Wouldn't you rather your partner be begging you for more rather than telling you that it's too much and to stop?

In addition to size, decide whether you want something realistic or a bit more fantastical. Some folks think a dildo that looks like a unicorn horn is delightful, while others want something that looks like a penis.

There's no perfect dildo for everyone, but making sure you and your partner are on the same page around size and appearance will make everyone happier. Shape is important, too; some dildos are curved for G-spot stimulation, but that might not feel good, based on the type of stimulation the person being penetrated likes. Communicate! Some dildos come with a removable vibrating bullet; if the toy you desire doesn't have one, you can buy one and tuck it into your harness.

Another option is a double-ended dildo. The original ones were useless to most women because two women's bodies together don't function in a straight line; these look more like dildo javelins than dildos designed to help people get off. Luckily, some sex toy manufactures realized this, and they've created new double-ended dildos. They're two differently shaped dildos stuck together. Place one end in your vagina (or anus), and using your Kegel muscles to hold it, put the other end in your partner (using lube), and go!

Sex toys are not regulated by the FDA, and some sex toys contain materials that aren't body-safe. These materials, called phthalates, are rubber softeners and are dangerous enough to be outlawed in children's toys. It's recommended that you choose sex toys that are phthalate-free. One way to do this is to buy only 100 percent silicone. If you already have a dildo that's made of another material that's not body-safe, use a condom on it during sex to protect you both.

Make sure your harness and cock fit well together, and try the set on and fit it to your body before it's time for the grand reveal. Adjust the straps for comfort, and figure out where you'd like the dildo to sit; try out a few places and decide what works best for you. Then practice getting in and out of it by yourself. This will help build your confidence for when it's time to slip it on in the middle of sexy time.

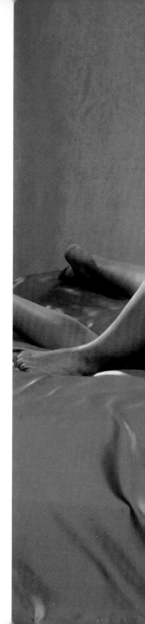

Not Your Mother's Missionary

One woman is wearing a strap-on harness and dildo. The receiving partner is on the bed, lying on her back with legs spread either flat out or bent at the knee with feet on the bed. She's being penetrated by her partner, who is on her knees. This seems simple, but you can mix it up by placing pillows under the woman lying down to change up the angles, by adding sex toys, or by having the kneeling partner also kiss and stimulate her partner's nipples.

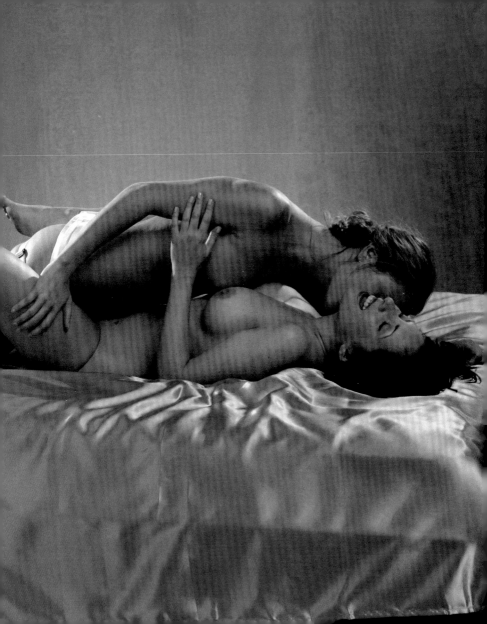

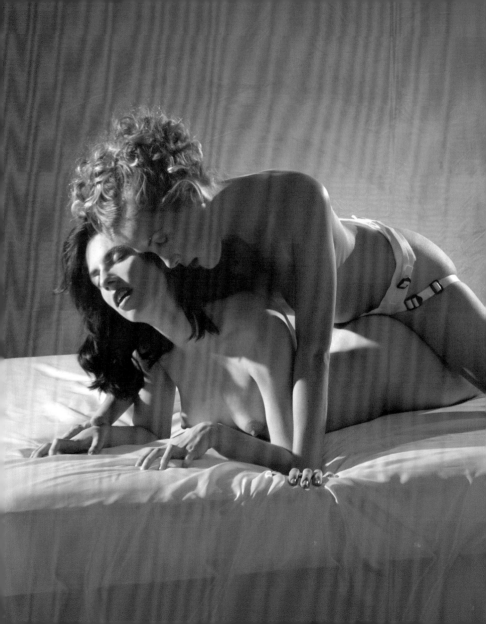

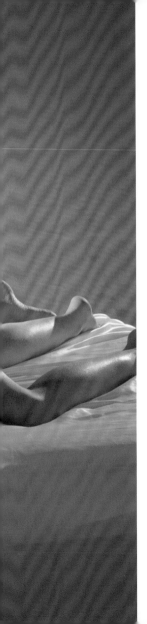

Full-Body Friction

A great position for those who love skin-on-skin contact! The woman receiving penetration is lying on the bed, on her stomach; she can use her elbows to hold her up or be flat on her chest, as she prefers. Her partner is strapped-on and is gently lying on top of her, sliding into either her vagina or anus, slowly working her way to a deeper and more intense penetration. Add some hair pulling or even a blindfold to spice up this position more, and a pillow under the penetratee's hips can change the angle!

That's a Wrap!

Similar to Not Your Mother's Missionary, in this position the receiver has her legs wrapped around the waist of her partner, who is penetrating her with the strap-on. This can help provide deeper sensation and also allow the woman being penetrated to control the depth of penetration to what feels good to her. Add a vibrator to get some extra clitoral stimulation.

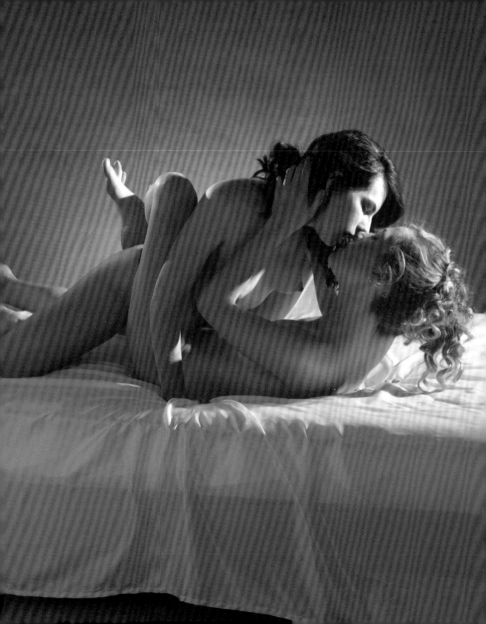

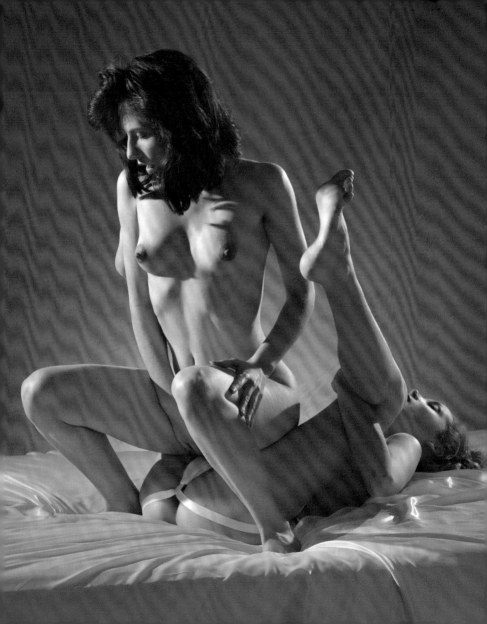

Snap, Crackle, POP!

Designed only for those with increased flexibility and dexterity, this position really takes strap-on sex to new levels. The woman who is strapped-on is lying on her back, legs spread, and supporting her knees as she pulls them to her chest. Her partner is squatting, facing away from her, riding the dildo and harness in a reverse cowgirl style. Definitely a position for the bucket list!

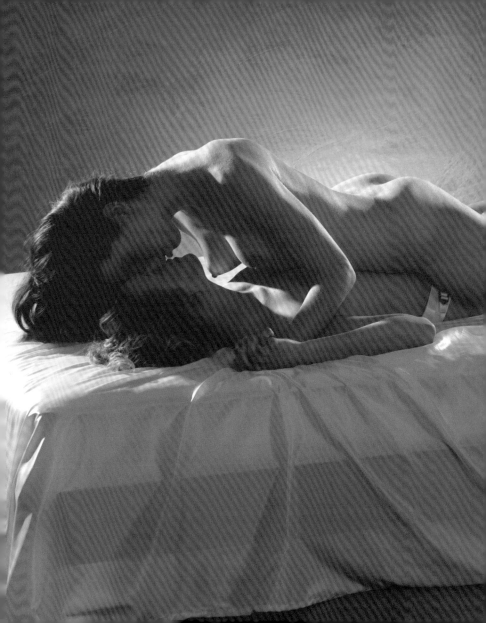

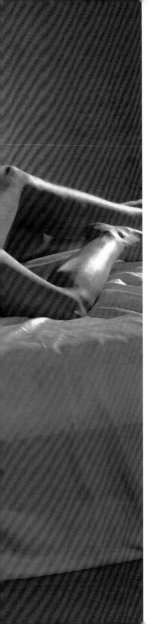

Intertwined Intimacy

Specifically for those who want to lock eyes with their lover during sex, this position allows for eye contact, skin on skin, and even intense hand-holding. Similar to a traditional woman-on-top-style position, in this move, the woman wearing the harness and dildo is lying on the bed, but her legs can be either bent or stretched out. Her partner is riding her, but leans forward to allow for her knees to be slightly spread on either side of the bottom woman's hips.

Blossoming Lotus

One woman is lying on her back on the bed with her legs doing a split in the air (she can reach out and hold her ankles open if it makes it easier). Her partner, wearing a harness and dildo, is kneeling between her legs, facing her, penetrating her while maintaining eye contact. This can provide a deeper penetration, and sometimes placing pillows under the receiving partner can change the angle of penetration for a different sensation.

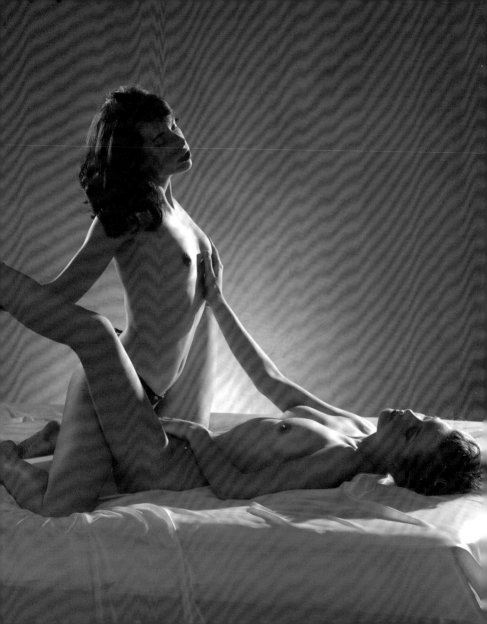

Sidesaddle

This is a missionarylike position, but with a bit of a twist...literally! The woman receiving the penetration is on her back with her legs bent up, and twisted to the side at her waist. A position like this then allows the woman who is strapped-on to kneel and enter from behind at a whole other angle, almost like rear entry, but while still letting them both maintain eye contact the whole time. The woman who is twisted can rest her legs on her partner's back, or can bring them up toward her lips for a little foot fetish action!

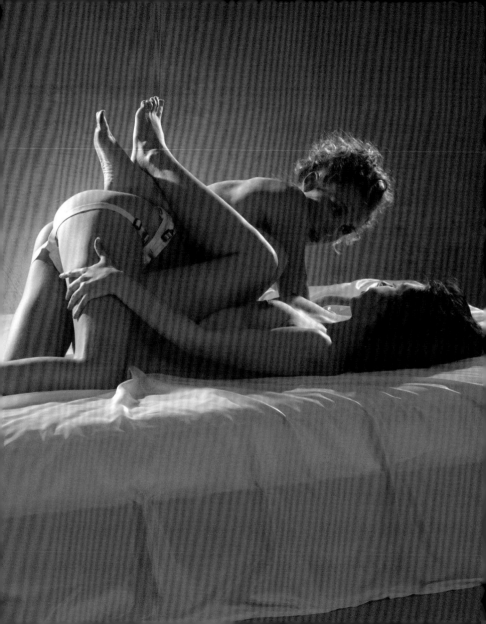

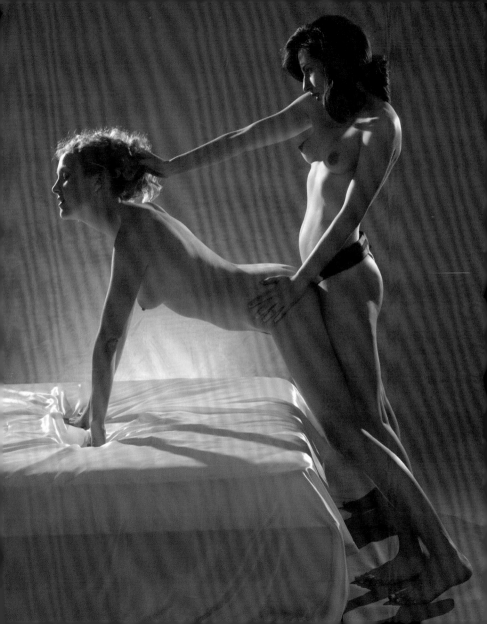

Bend Over, Baby

The receiver is standing at the edge of the bed, bent over, supporting herself on the bed with her hands, elbows, or forearms. Her partner is behind her, wearing a harness and dildo, penetrating her. The giver can have her hand wrapped in the hair of the receiver, or be reaching around to stimulate her nipples. The person bent over can reach down and play with herself or even use a vibrator to help stimulate her clitoris.

Ride 'Em Hard!

Similar to the traditional "cowgirl" position, this position has the partner wearing the strap-on lying on her back on the bed, while the receiver either kneels or squats with her legs on either side, facing her partner. The women can stimulate each other's breasts, nipples, and even vulvar regions while in this position, and provide support for the rider as needed. The rider can choose the angle and depth of penetration for whatever feels best to her. For additional comfort, place pillows under the rider's knees and/or the prone partner's neck.

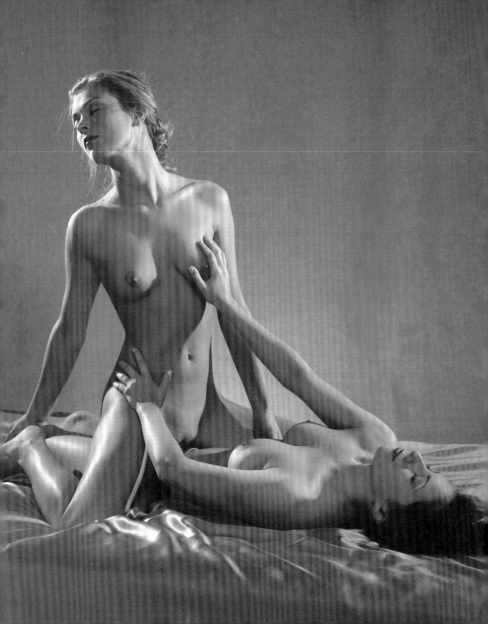

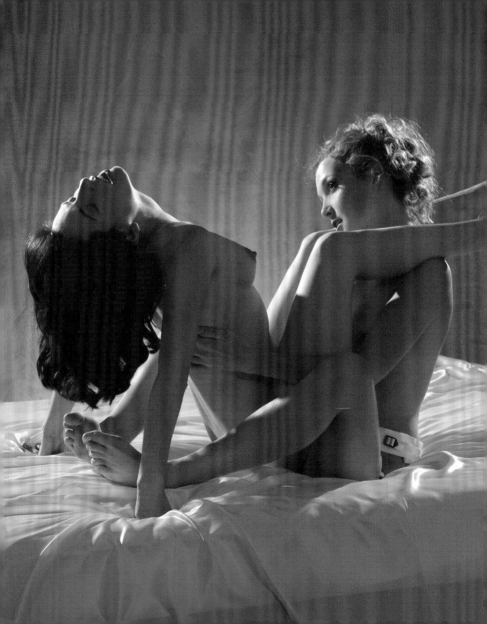

Heels over Head

A position that allows for both physical closeness and continuous eye contact, this is designed for a receiver who is a bit more flexible. With the partner wearing the harness and dildo sitting on the bed with her feet together and knees open, the woman getting penetrated comes close to her, placing her feet and knees over her partner's shoulders while supporting her torso with her arms behind her. Once connected, they can rock back and forth for additional stimulation.

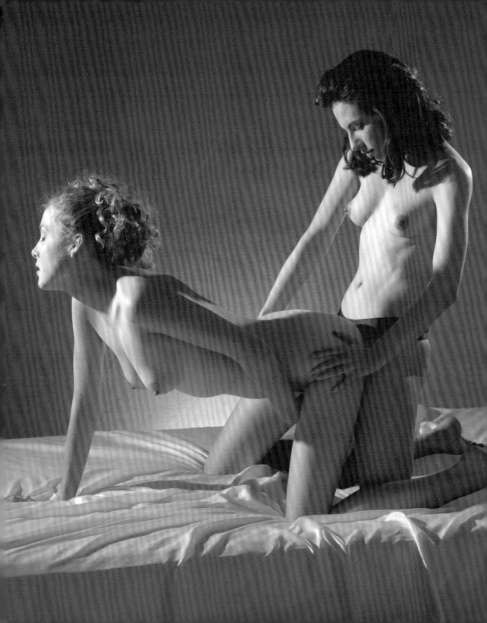

The Cat's Meow

The receiving woman is on her hands and knees (in a traditional doggy-style position) with her back arched, chest forward, and hips up and back (like "cow" in cat-cow pose in yoga). Her partner is behind her wearing a strap-on, penetrating her vaginally. The receiver has one hand reaching back underneath her to stimulate her clit. Pillows can be placed under either or both partners' knees to add more comfort if needed.

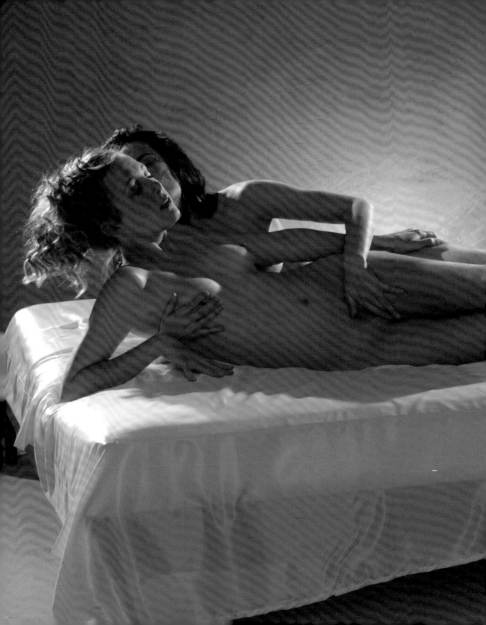

Big Spoon and Little Spoon

Both women are in a spooning position, with the woman in back wearing a harness and dildo that is vaginally penetrating her partner. Both of them have their legs straightened (so they look like two spoons in a drawer), and the woman wearing the strap-on can be kissing or biting the receiver's neck, as well as reaching around to stimulate her nipples, clitoris, and so on.

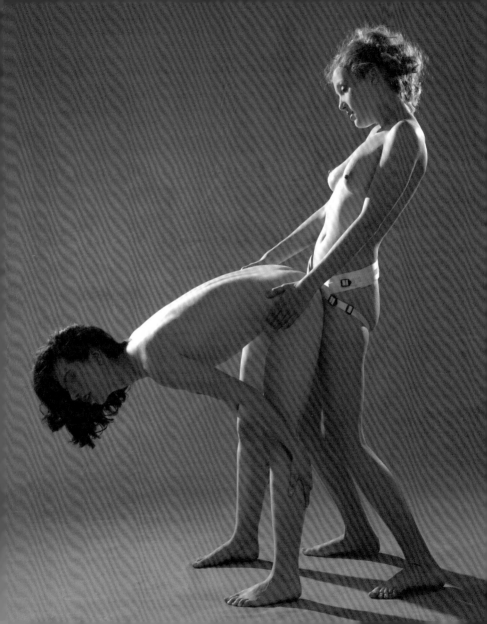

Acrobatic Angles

Similar to good ol' doggy-style, this position offers even deeper penetration as well as a great stretch for both parties involved. The woman in back is strapped-on, supporting her partner by holding onto her waist. Her partner is in front, being penetrated from behind while bending forward, almost in half. She can either support herself by placing her hands on the floor, or can grab or wrap her arms around her knees to steady herself a bit.

The Randy Reach

The woman receiving is on her knees and her forearms or hands, leaning forward, forming a triangle with her body and the bed. Her partner is behind her, wearing a strap-on, and is on her knees, penetrating her lover vaginally. Placing a pillow beneath either or both partners' knees can make things more comfortable. This would be a great position to place a blindfold or wrist restraints on the receiving partner if she might like to experiment with that.

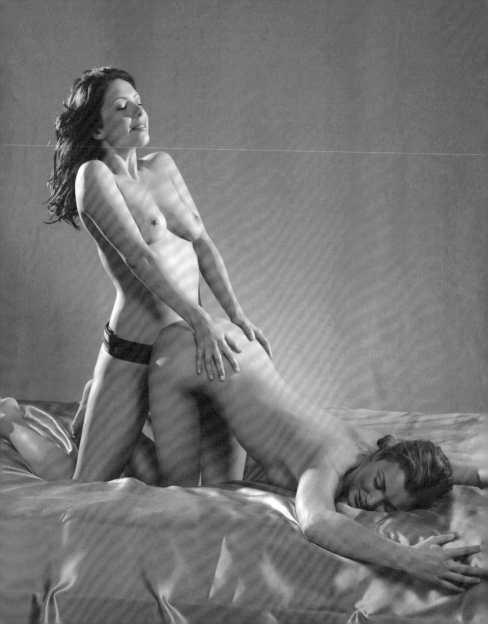

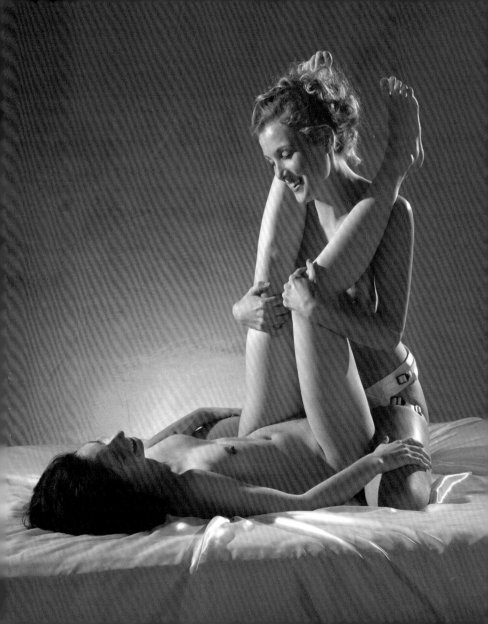

Control Tower

The woman who will be receiving the penetration is lying on her back, her legs up in the air forming an L shape with her body. Her partner is strapped-on, and is kneeling, allowing the first woman's legs to rest on her while she penetrates her. A great position that allows the woman being penetrated to control of depth as she moves her legs closer to or farther from her partner, or even by bending at the knees. Also allows for great eye contact!

The Executive

Using a chair, the partner who is wearing the harness and dildo sits comfortably as her partner straddles her or even squats over her, rocking back and forth or up and down for different feelings of penetration. The sitting partner should support the riding partner so that there are no falls; if this looks fun but you are worried, try a similar style of position but on the floor or bed (like Intertwined Intimacy).

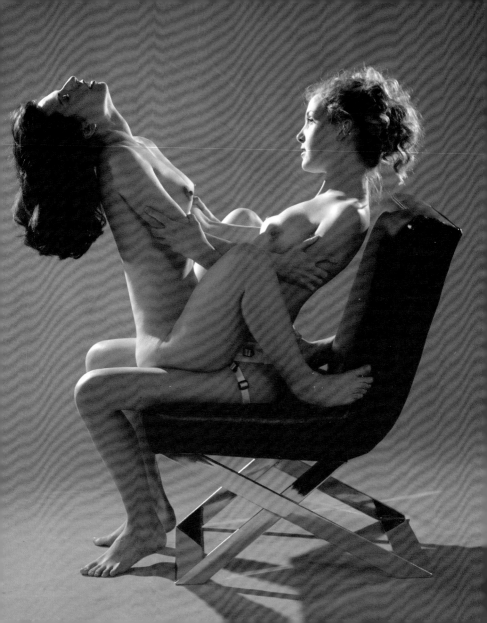

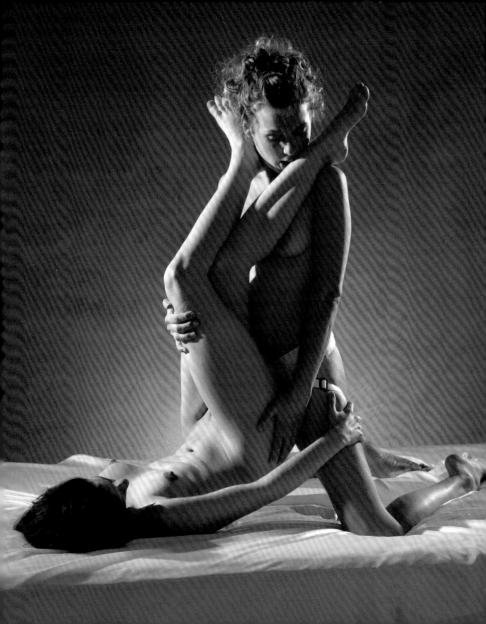

X Marks the Spot

The receiving woman is on her back with her crossed legs in the air and balanced on her partner's shoulders as she is being penetrated. She can either support herself with core strength or use her arms or some pillows to help support her hips. This is a similar position to Blast Off, but with the woman who is being penetrated crossing her legs for a whole new type of stimulation. It allows for deeper penetration while maintaining the option of eye contact, and has some foot loving built in for those who enjoy toes!

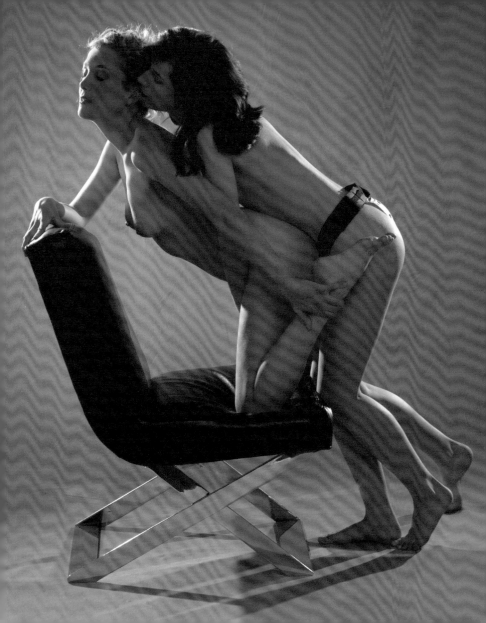

Spider Woman

One woman is bent over the bed or a chair and is being vaginally penetrated by her partner standing behind her, who is wearing a harness and dildo. The woman bent over is standing on only one leg, and the other leg is up, foot on the bed (bent at the knee), allowing her penetrating partner to stimulate her vulva during sex. The partner wearing the strap-on can reach down or around to help play with the receiving partner's clitoris, or that woman can help stimulate herself.

Crouching Cowgirl

Similar in many ways to the more traditional cowgirl position, in this position the woman who is strapped-on is lying on the bed on her back (use pillows under her hips to change the angle if you'd like to mix things up). Her partner, with one leg on either side of the lying partner's hips, is squatting over her, allowing her to control the depth and speed of the penetration. This could be a fun position for bondage or a blindfold, or even adding a vibrator or two!

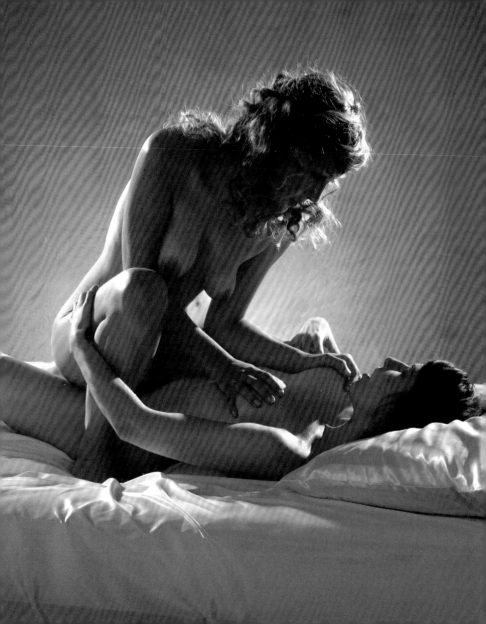

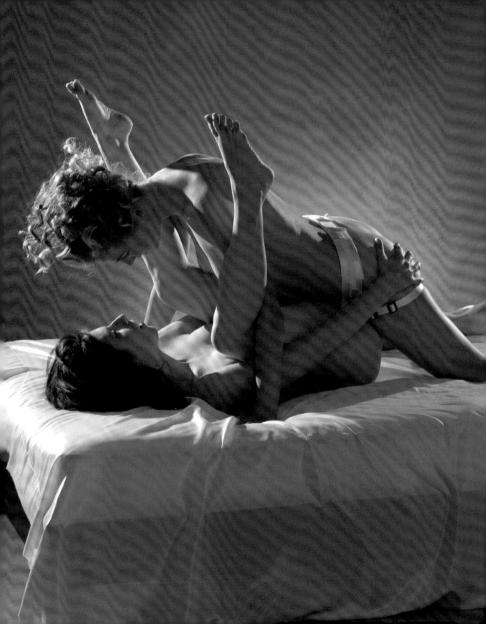

Folded Fornication

A bit like a more traditional missionary, this position has the added bonus of much deeper penetration. The woman being penetrated is lying on her back on the bed, her knees bent up toward her chest, and she can further support this position by holding onto her knees, or she can reach down to connect with the other woman. Her partner is then between her legs (either kneeling or on bent knees with more straightened legs), penetrating her. If a pillow is added under the receiving partner's hips, this can allow for even deeper penetration at a new angle if so desired.

Blast Off

The woman wearing a harness and dildo is on her knees on the bed. Her partner is lying on the bed on her back. She places her feet on the kneeling partner's shoulders and supports her lower back with her hands or multiple pillows. The kneeling partner penetrates her vaginally and helps support the partner on her back by holding her hips.

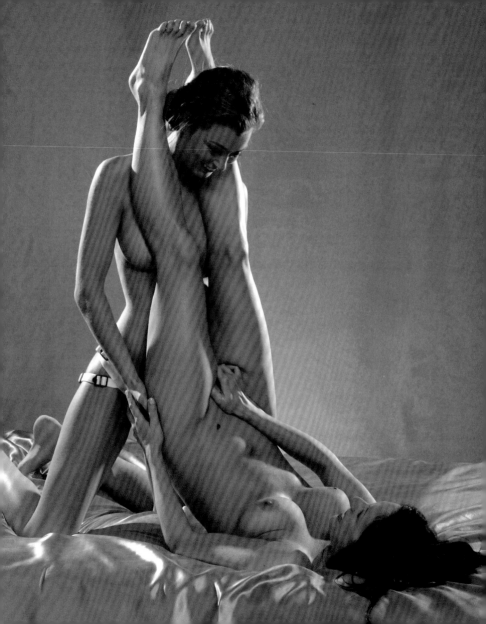

On Your Knees, Please

Using a stable, freestanding (not rocking) chair, one woman is kneeling on the seat of the chair, supporting herself with chair's back. Her partner is wearing a harness and dildo and has come up behind her to penetrate her. The kneeling woman can spread her legs slightly and bend forward as much as she can to increase the depth of penetration, while the standing partner can support her by holding onto her hips.

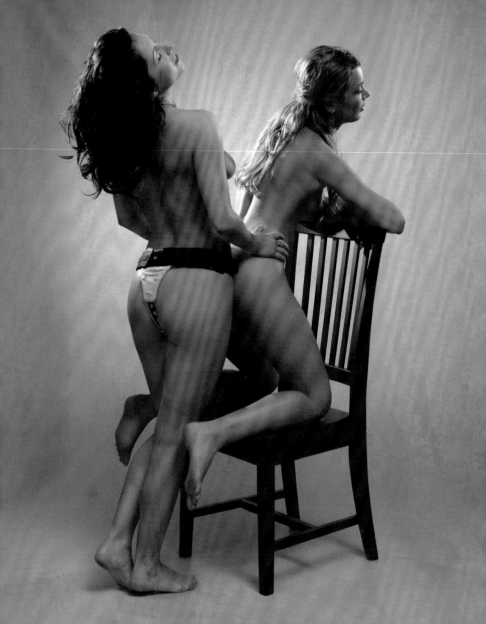

Bending toward Bliss

One woman starts by lying on her back on the bed while wearing a harness and dildo, and the other woman straddles her on her knees, facing the end of the bed as she places the dildo inside her. The kneeling woman then lies back onto her partner, so the penetrating partner can stimulate her nipples and even reach down to provide clitoral stimulation if she would like. Pillows under the kneeling partner's knees can help make this more comfortable.

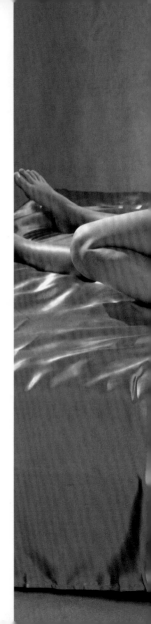

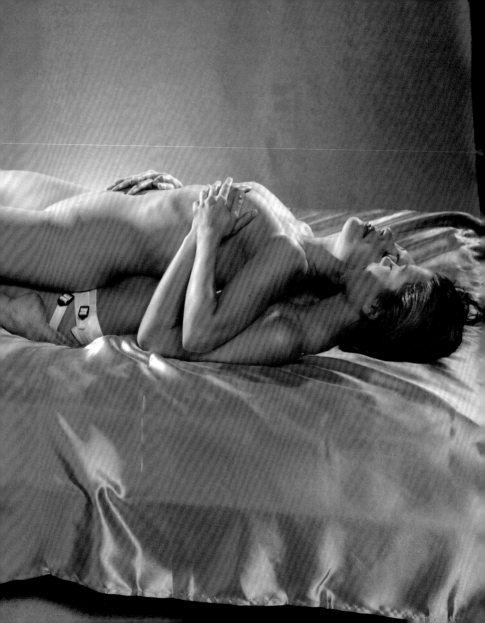

Puzzle Pieces

One woman is wearing a harness and dildo, sitting cross-legged or in a butterfly position (knees bent, bottoms of feet touching) on the bed or floor. Her partner then straddles her, placing the dildo inside her, and wrapping her legs around her until they fit together comfortably. Don't do this near the edge of the bed, as it can be a bit precarious. It can help if one or both partners use their hands on the bed or wall for extra balance. This position is less for thrusting than it is for the rotating of hips and doing Kegel exercises.

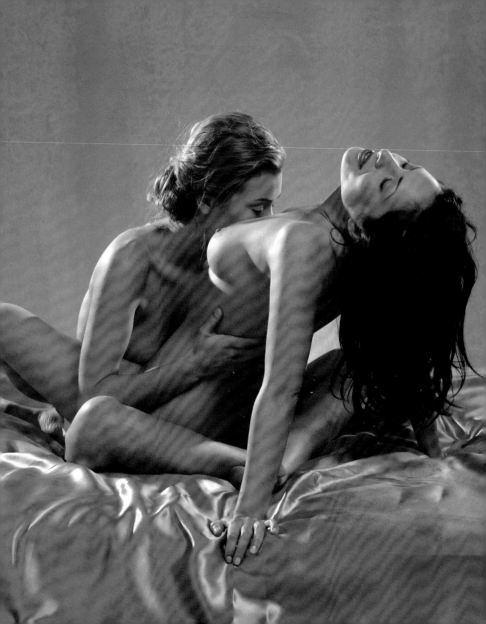

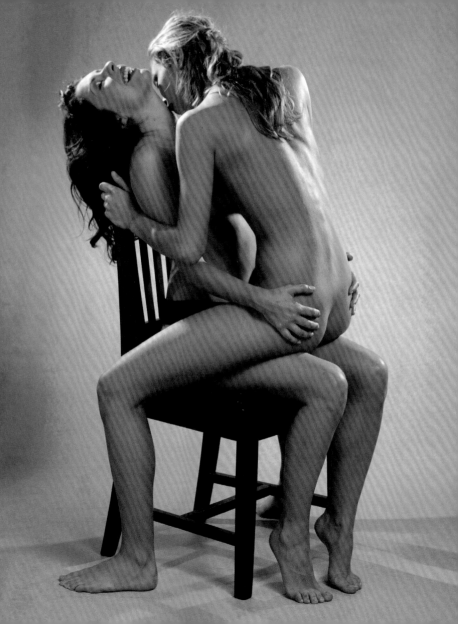

The Strap-On Straddle

One partner has strapped on a harness and dildo and is sitting in a stable chair with her legs together. Her partner then straddles her, placing the dildo inside her. Because they're facing each other, they can use their arms not only to support each other but also to stimulate each other's nipples, vulvas, and so on. Additionally, they can kiss, bite, and whatever else feels good to them.

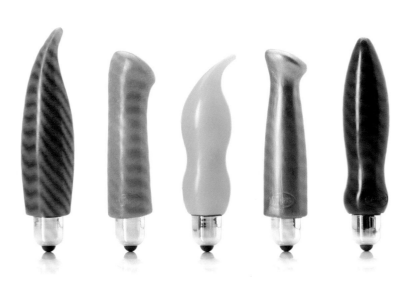

TOYING AROUND

Sex toys have been around almost as long as humans have. No fooling: there have been dildos found made out of granite that come from prehistoric times. But in the last century or so, society has made significant advances in the field of sex toys designed solely for increasing sexual pleasure. In the late 1990s and early 2000s, the Rabbit vibrator made its debut on *Sex and the City*, causing hordes of women to descend on sex toy stores across the U.S. Everyone and their sister had a joke about double-ended dildos, butt plugs, or what have you. They've become a standard part of our conversation. From vibrators to butt plugs, dildos to cock rings, a sex toys is available for pretty much every sexy activity you can think of.

Unfortunately, there's sometimes a taboo in some groups about the use of sex toys, especially with a partner, and sadly, that can leave people feeling scared, intimidated, or guilty about wanting to bring these vehicles of sexual pleasure into the bedroom or wherever their sexual experiences are taking place. But as our culture continues to evolve and we work to normalize the importance of sexual pleasure, sex toys are losing some of their stigma. Today, for many people, sex toys have become household objects, and some of them even have their own names. I'm not saying that you have to love sex toys to have amazing sex—they aren't for everyone. That said, for many, sex toys are a fun way to put a little more pizzazz into their sex life or to try new and adventurous activities.

So, you've decided to add some toys to your bedroom routine? Fabulous! But before you run down the street to your friendly neighborhood sex toy retailer, just stop for a moment and think. Does your partner like surprises? Have you discussed the possible use of sex toys before? If the answer to either of these questions is no, it might be a good idea to chat her up about purchasing an item of the sex toy variety. In fact, for many couples, going shopping for the new toy together (either online or by visiting a store) is a great way to pick out a toy that both of you are comfortable with and that both of you will like. This way, it's not just one of you picking out a toy and showing it to the other: you both have a vested interest in the toy since it was one that got you both excited. Now, if you're single and want to invest in a harness and dildo, or beloved vibrator, so that you're prepared for the next lady who wants to get down and dirty, then more power to you!

There's absolutely no shame in owning and/or using a sex toy (or many sex toys). Think of it in comparison to your kitchen supplies or the tools in your workshop. Can you roll dough by hand? Sure, but it's nice to have a rolling pin, and even a dough press to mix things up.

Can you cut some wood by hand, and drill holes for screws manually? Absolutely, but a power saw and an electric drill can make your life a little more fun at times. It's great to have a variety of tools available to get the job done when you want, as well as have the ability to use manual labor.

Recent studies have shown that anywhere from 50 to 75 percent of women use or have used sex toys, and somewhere from 33 to 50 percent of men have done the same. That's a lot of people welcoming toys into their sex lives. Television shows have normalized sex toys for masturbation, and mainstream magazines talk about using sex toys along with your partner on a regular basis. It might be a little bit over the top to make the blanket statement that everyone's doing it, and it's important to remember that sex toys aren't the right fit for everyone. But using sex toys is becoming mainstream in our society, and doing so can add a lot of fun new dimensions to your sex life!

Helping Hand

Toys are good for so much more than "just" stimulation and penetration alone. In this position, the giver of oral delight is also using a vibrator or a dildo to get some extra action for her partner, in addition to her talented tongue. Take whatever position already works best, and then add a little outside helper (vibrator, dildo, paddle; you name it) to really take her over the world and back again! Plus, if oral sex is going to last for a long time, this concept provides the giver with some much needed refresher breaks.

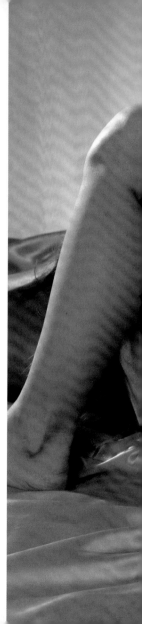

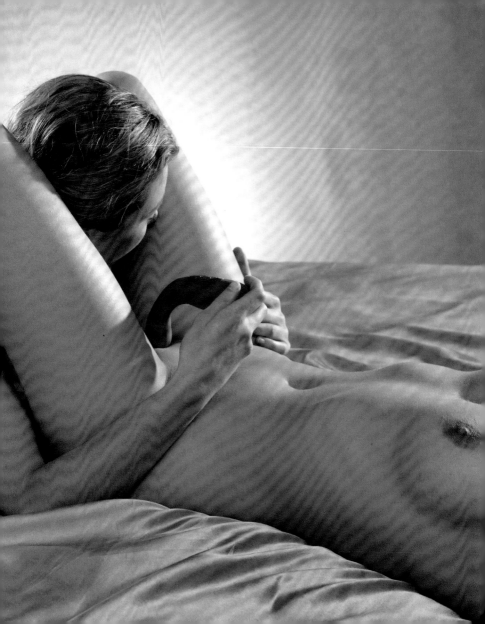

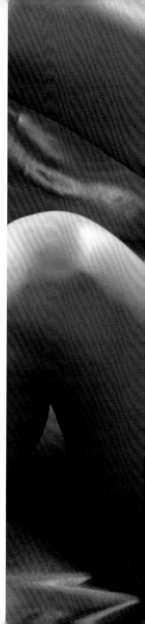

Criss-Cross

Both women are lying on the bed on their backs, or one can be propped up on her elbow or her side so that they can look at each other and enjoy the action. Their legs are slightly spread and can bend at the knee, being as close to each other as feels comfortable. Each is holding her partner's favorite vibrator or dildo and is reaching across her own body to stimulate the other. This is a great way for each partner to learn how the other likes to be touched and to practice the safer-sex technique of mutual masturbation where no body fluids are shared.

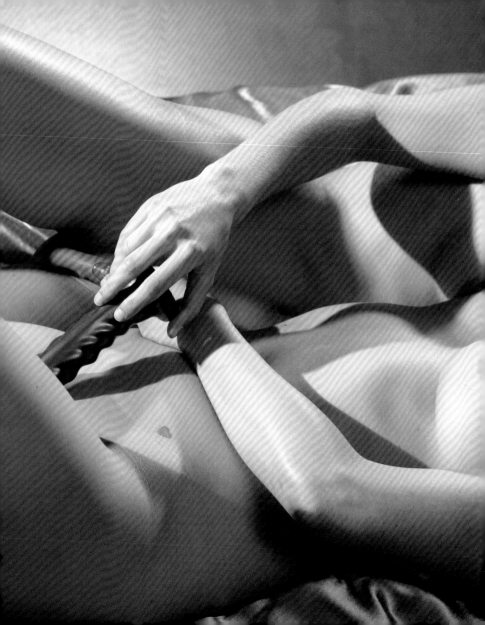

Captivating Control

Both women are standing up, with one standing behind the other. The woman in front can stimulate her own breasts and nipples or reach behind her to touch and feel connected with her partner. The woman standing behind reaches around to stimulate her partner's vulva with a vibrator. If she wants, she can also have her own vibrator so they are getting dual stimulation.

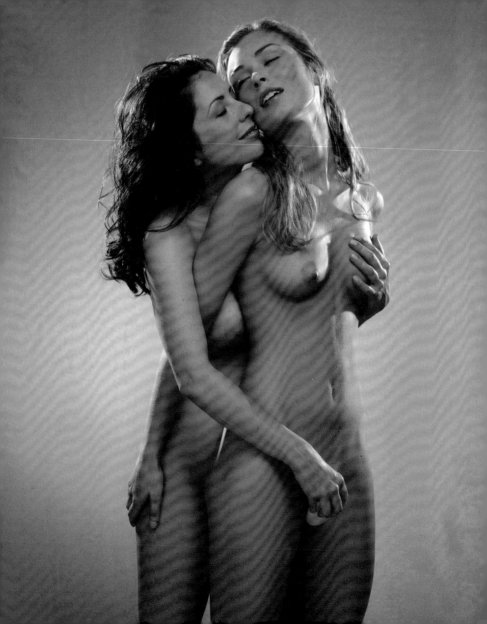

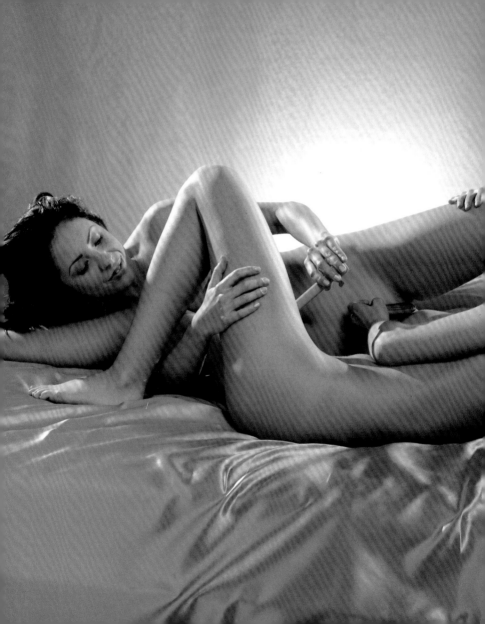

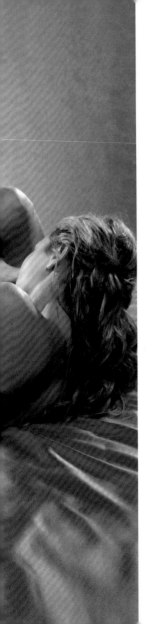

Good Vibes

Both women are on the bed in almost a traditional 69 position, except the woman on the bottom has her legs spread more, and the woman on top is more on her hands and knees, and neither of their heads are between each other's legs. Instead, they each have a vibrator and are using them to stimulate each other's vulvas. The woman on top can support her body weight with her non-toy-holding hand.

233

The Rocking Chair

One woman is sitting on a stable (non-rocking) chair with her feet firmly on the floor. The other woman faces her and straddles both her and the chair. The woman sitting on the chair now licks, nips, and stimulates the straddling woman's nipples while stabilizing her, putting her hands on or around her waist. The straddling woman uses a vibrator to stimulate her clitoris and labia. With the appropriate vibrator (or vibrators!), they can stimulate each other simultaneously!

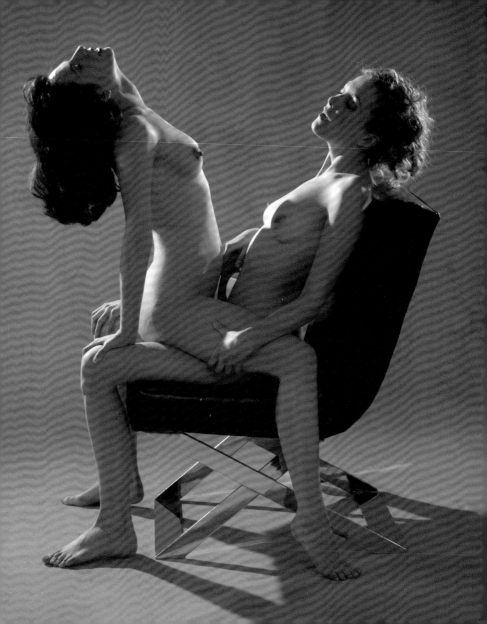

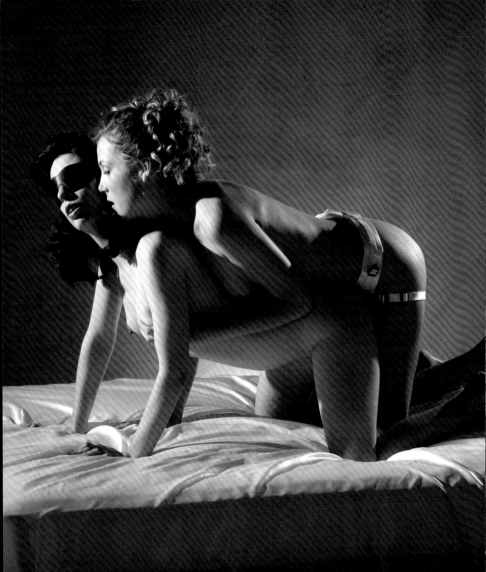

Fade to Black

One woman is on her hands and knees on the bed, wearing a blindfold. Her partner is kneeling behind her, leaning forward so her breasts are pressed against her partner's back, and the top partner is using both of her hands to stimulate the blindfolded woman's nipples and breasts. This could also be a great way to bring nipple clamps into play; make sure you start light and work your way up.

Whoa There

Whatever activity you're doing, a blindfold can help increase the other sensations. And if you and your partner have discussed playing around with hair pulling, spanking, and so on, the blindfold can help ramp up the anticipation of these things happening. Try it out, see how each of you likes it, and decide if it works for you at all.

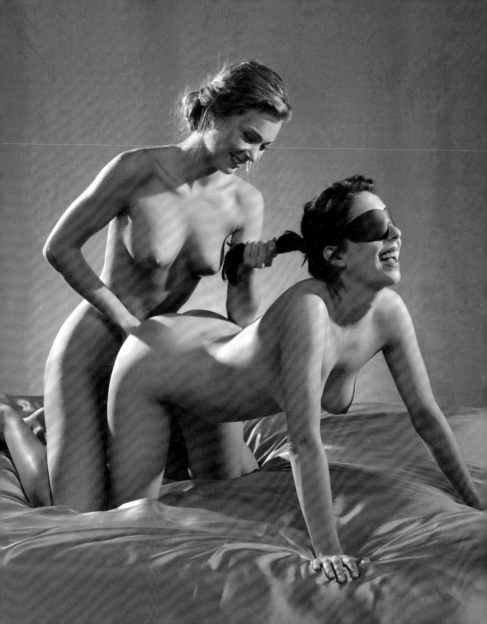

WRAPPING IT UP

TOOL TIME:
Talking Toys

Whether or not you choose to add toys to your repertoire, it's good to have some info about toys for adults.

Decades ago, a myth seemed to gain traction that if women use sex toys, particularly vibrators, they'll become addicted to their toy and never again want to have sex with another human. Guess what? It's just that: a myth. There have been absolutely no case studies of women wanting to marry, much less date or move in with, their sex toy of choice. Why not, since they can be so sexually pleasurable? It's because vibrators don't cuddle, they don't help with chores, they're poor conversation starters, and they certainly don't have multiple digits and a tongue.

Well, then, one might ask why even use toys if they can't kiss you or bring home the bacon? Because what they can do is help you (and your partner) reach fabulous orgasms, explore new and exciting activities, and add a new dimension to your sex life, alone or together.

Now, it's true that some women might become attached to the sensation of a toy (or a specific type of stimulation provided by a human partner), or they may wind up feeling a bit desensitized after using the same toy for a longer period of time. But the solution is easy—stop using the toy for a week or two (or longer if needed), and your body will return to where it was. No need for reparative therapy or anything hard core like that. Let your body reset, and then you can explore the same or new sensations offered either by toys or by your partner. Problem solved.

One of the most basic, original, and likely best-known sex toys is, of course, the vivacious vibrator. Vibrators come in all sorts of shapes, sizes, colors, patterns, and styles. There are three distinct types: those for internal (vaginal or sometimes anal) stimulation, those for external (usually clitoral, occasionally anal) stimulation, and those that provide dual stimulation (usually of both the clitoris and vagina; the infamous Rabbit is the best-known example of the dual-stimulation type of toy). Some women will want one from each category, while others know that they prefer clitoral vibrators and fingers or dildos inside, or that dual stimulators just don't work for them. There's no right or wrong answer on which style of stimulation is best for women overall.

Within each of these categories, you can find those powered by batteries, those that are rechargeable, and of course, a few that still plug into the wall. In the last category, the most well-known is the Hitachi Magic Wand vibrator (originally designed as a vibrating massager), which is sometimes called the Cadillac of vibrators. Figure out which works best for you. Will you remember to charge a rechargeable vibrator, or will you want to use it only to find out it's dead? Are you ready to invest in the batteries needed (keep in mind some vibrators use watch batteries, which are harder to find and more expensive to replace than your average AA or AAA batteries) to keep you and your partner rumbling along? Is your bed near an electrical outlet, or does your power frequently cut out? All things to consider.

How to use them? I hope you'll be able to experiment with what you enjoy by yourself, but sometimes it can get a little complicated. If you're using a vibrator with your partner, make sure she gets in on the action. While the vibrator is . . . well . . . vibing, the other partner can play with the vibrator-receiver's nipples, give lots of sweet kisses, use her fingers for manual stimulation, or even take control of the toy. Just because you've brought the toy into your playtime doesn't mean that you have to keep the toy going throughout. It's okay to bring the vibe into play for a little bit, and then tag team it out when the other partner wants to use some more manual, oral, or other action. You can also make good use of an external vibrator while one partner (or both) are in the middle of oral sex, penetration, friction play, and so on. Just think about where the clits will be, and if there's room, slide a vibrator between the bodies to give a little boost in clitoral stimulation.

Yet another option is to place an internal-stimulation vibrator inside one partner's vagina, buzzing away while she goes down on, manually stimulates, or uses a toy to penetrate her partner. Just because you're being the giver in a sexual situation doesn't mean you don't get to have some physical pleasure happening at the same time! For the receiver, some like the feeling of being full, and while that can be achieved by a non-vibrating dildo (as I discuss shortly), some people really like the feeling of internal vibrators. Just remember that with sex toys, lube is love. Don't forget to add lube for any toy action, as a toy without lube can create extra drag on the skin, and that likely will not feel good.

As with all toys, it's highly recommended that you stay away from vibrators (and really, all sex toys) that are made of jelly rubber (also called gelée and Sil-a-Gel). This material contains phthalates, which are not good for your body and are actually regulated in children's toys. Because sex toys don't go through the FDA approval process, they can pretty much contain anything, and not much research has been done on the materials. The studies that have been done show that phthalates can leach from the toys into vaginal and anal tissue, causing irritation, allergic relation, and potentially cancer. Look for toys made of hard plastic, TPR (thermoplastic rubber), elastomer, glass, wood, metal, and medical-grade silicone to make sure you're getting something that's okay for you health-wise. If you're in love with a jelly toy or don't have the finances to get something new, please consider using a condom over the toy to protect your body from phthalates. Some companies making body-friendly vibrators in a variety of shapes, styles, colors, designs, and sizes are LELO, Je Joue, Jimmy Jane, Tantus, Vibratex, Big Teaze, Fun Factory, Love Honey, and OhMiBod.

One nice thing about vibrators (or any toy) made out of medical-grade silicone (or metal, ceramic, or glass) is that you can sterilize them by wiping them down with a 10 percent bleach solution and washing them off (if they're toys that don't vibrate, you can also boil them for three to five minutes, or put them on the top shelf of your dishwasher). Why does it matter if you sterilize them? Because you can then safely use them with multiple partners without worrying about transmitting bacteria, urinary tract infections, sexually transmitted infections, and so on. And if you use a toy to stimulate your anus, or penetrate it, you'll need to sterilize it (or use a condom) before you can use it again vaginally. So be picky with your materials; supply is based on consumer demand. If we demand better-quality sex toys by only purchasing ones that are safe for our bodies, the companies will then make more body-friendly sex toys. Ta-da!

Let's move on to dildos! For the most part, dildos are designed for either filling the vagina or being thrust in and out of the vagina (some dildos are also anal friendly, but only if they have a base that's wider than the rest of the toy—check out the anal section for more info on this!). Add a little bit of water-based lubricant to keep things sliding smoothly, and either partner can help operate the dildo throughout all types of sexual experiences. While many people think dildos are only for use with strap-on play (and don't worry; if that's your thing, there's a whole section on that), you can also use dildos during oral sex, as part of manual stimulation, during mutual masturbation, and more.

Dildos, like most sex toys, come in all sorts of shapes, sizes, materials, colors, realness versus not-realness, and so on. There are thinner dildos designed for anal play, medium dildos designed for all types of play, and of course, some larger dildos that are perfect for those size queens who enjoy feeling really full. Most dildos don't vibrate, but some have a bullet vibrator in their base (that can be taken out for cleaning) to add a little vibration action to your playtime. You can also find double-ended dildos, harness-friendly dildos, unicorn horn look-a-like dildos, and many other options. Check out the strap-on section to learn more about different types of dildos, choosing a dildo, good materials for dildos, and more!

Now let's discuss toys that aren't geared just for your vulva and your anus. One such item could potentially be considered a sex toy, but is more of a delightful sex-cessory. Using this can help you optimize your sensations during your sexual experiences. What are we talking about? Blindfolds, of course! Why are they so fabulous? Because when you take away one sensation (in this case, your sight), you increase the efficacy of your other senses, and so in this case smell, taste, sound, and touch are that much more intense. When it comes to blindfolds, you have a few options: there are gorgeous satin, leather, and other types of blindfolds that you can purchase to match your boudoir, or you can use a scarf, tie, or other such items wrapped around your head. In addition to the increase in your sense of touch, you can play with your other senses by experimenting with food, sexy and sensual music, and scented candles or incense. This can ramp up the experience for the person wearing the blindfold, and if she doesn't like the feeling, she can always remove it easily and quickly.

Yet another sex toy that focuses on other fabulous body parts is nipple clamps. Now, for some people, these might seem a little intimidating or scary. Not to worry. The different types of clamps you can purchase can go from mild to wild, and everywhere in between. Whatever the size of your nipples, whether or not they're pierced, clamps can work on any type of nipples. You can find oodles of nipple clamps online or at your local toy store, including tweezer clamps, alligator clamps, and clover clamps, with their intensity increasing in that order. If you're nipple clamp newbies, it would probably be best to start with tweezer clamps, because they're easy to adjust and don't get too tight. If you find that they don't provide enough sensation for you or your partner, then feel free to step up to alligator or even clover clamps. If you're not ready to go out and buy your own set of nice nipple clamps, wooden clothespins are a worthy substitute, and they can be loosened (if they feel too tight) by placing rubber bands around the tips. As with all sensation things, remember to start easy and work your way up, and don't leave nipple clamps or clothespins on for more than about 20 minutes. Fair warning: they usually hurt a bit coming off as well, so keep that in mind before you decide to remove them. If all of this sounds like too much, there are also superlightweight vibrating nipple clamps, and even nipple pumps that provide lots of fun sensation but without any amount of "ouch!"

In addition to blindfolds and nipple clamps, it can be fun to add a little kinky play to your bedroom playtime. Trying out a bit of bondage can go a long way in keeping the spice in your sex life. Please remember to be careful about using metal handcuffs (real or play ones), as metal pressing against moving wrists can cause nerve damage in some folks. Never fear though—sex-friendly wrist restraints and ankle restrains can be a fun, simple, and comfortable way to keep either the giver or receiver still as you take turns offering each other all types of naughty enjoyment. You can just bind your partner with wrist or ankle cuffs, or you can use the variety of nylon webbing under-bed restraint systems designed for holding your partner down or in one place without having to renovate your bedroom or drill hooks into the walls.

Another option you can experiment with is using scarves or ties, but please remember these tend to get tighter and tighter as they are pulled on (as do pantyhose or nylons!), so it's worth having a pair of medical shears or safety scissors in case any knots or ties get too tight. If anyone's hands get cold or turn blue, make sure to take the bondage off right away. Remember to start slow and work your way up; it's always more exciting to add more and more fun things to your time together than to scare your lover off by showing up with an entire working dungeon without discussing it first! Keep in mind that if someone's tied up, you probably don't want to also have her gagged, as she'll be unable to tell you (or for you to tell her) if something's hurting and not working right. So while stuffing your panties in someone's mouth might be hot in your dreams, it might be more realistic to tell her to keep her mouth shut (and to playfully punish her when she doesn't) than it would be to physically keep her quiet.

Sensation play, especially when used alongside blindfolds and bondage, can be incredibly enjoyable for either or both of you. Feather ticklers (designed for this purpose or purchased at a craft store) can feel fabulous, and even household items like basting brushes, toothpicks, hairbrushes, bathroom loofahs, and more can provide a variety of different and exciting sensations as they're lightly placed and moved over the skin while you and your partner enjoy each other. If one partner is blindfolded, the other can ask her to guess what toys are being used, and if one partner is tied up, the other can caringly torment and tickle her until she can't take it anymore. As with any and all power play, if the word "no" doesn't mean "no" anymore (like "oh no, no, that feels so intense, I just can't take it anymore" . . . when she really wants you to keep going), you both should decide on a new word that now means "no" when you're together, like "red," "halt," or "cantaloupe." This is also true of role-playing or real-life fantasies that involve power dynamics, as well as bondage, gagging, or any play that might need a word to indicate an ALL PLAY STOPS NOW type of limit. It's important to discuss new directions of sexual activity, toys, and so on with your partner instead of just springing them on her; when both of you have excitement and buy-in around the new things, you're sure to have a much more exciting time together!

SLIP 'N' SLIDE:
Loving Lube

Lube. Perhaps it conjures up an image of changing oil in your car, or maybe a steamier picture of someone rubbing oil all over her body. Regardless of what it brings to mind, lube is one of the most important parts of good sex. Seriously folks, lube is love. Say it, think it, memorize it, and use it. Lube can truly optimize your sex life.

Why lube? Why not! Lubrication is an integral part of sexy times, and it's clear to see why. Lubrication makes all kinds of touch feel better below the belt, both outside on the lips, clitoris, and hood, as well as inside the vagina or anus, whether you're using fingers, tongues, or toys. It helps reduce friction, which if you weren't aware, is something that most vulvas don't like unless there is lube involved. Really, test it out. Try some stroking without lube, and then add it, and do it again. In general, vulvas prefer slippery, slidey sensations to those that produce friction and drag.

That's not all, folks! Lube can help transmit all sorts of sensations better, which in turn may lower the amount of effort required of the person providing said sensations. If you're penetrating a partner, lube makes it easier and smoother to go in and out. And if penetration is part of the picture (either vaginally or anally), using lube can absolutely help prevent or reduce soreness, as well as prevent tearing of the delicate vaginal tissue. Clearly, lube is our friend.

Given that the majority of vulvas lubricate on their own, to one extent or another, with some tending to provide more natural lubrication than others, people may ask why additional lube is needed. Here's the deal: the amount of lube produced by a vulva doesn't always directly correlate to how turned on the person is; a person can be ready to jump her partner like a wild animal in heat, yet have little to no lubricant being produced naturally, while someone else may have a geyser of lubricant being produced by her vagina, yet her mind is more focused on which color nail polish to use than on sex. Because of this, we can't use lubrication amount as an indication of arousal. Instead, this is where communication comes in. Try asking your partner if she's interested in some sexy playtime, if she's turned on, and if she's ready for you to do deliciously dirty things to her. The answers she gives you are going to be a much better indication of whether she's ready for naughtiness than whether she's full of lubrication.

Even though most vulvas have the natural ability to lubricate, a whole bevy of things can affect natural lubrication, which results in a somewhat dried-out vagina (although clearly, vaginas are never completely dry; they retain moisture in their mucosal membrane constantly). What are these evils that dry out our beloved pussies? The list can include hormonal birth control (the patch, the pill, the ring, the Implanon, the shot, etc.), antihistamines (any allergy medication, both prescription and over-the-counter), and stress (which tends to affect anyone capable of breathing). Given that lesser or lack of lubrication can happen from any of these very common things, and the fact that sometimes sex sessions can last for hours on end, it's always good to have some vulva-friendly lube on hand.

What makes a lubricant vulva-friendly? Well, first of all, it shouldn't have any oil or petroleum product in the ingredient list. Think about your hands when you're washing dishes; if you get a layer of oil on them, water just beads up until you use a hard-core grease-cutting soap to clean up. Same goes for the vagina. If you put an oil-based lube (or lotion, or cooking oil, etc.) in the vaginal canal, it will coat the walls of the vagina. This is bad, because the vagina cleans itself through transudation, where fluid comes through the walls of the vagina, like an overfilled sponge. If you coat the walls with oil or oil-like substances, you prevent the vagina from cleaning itself. This means it's now more susceptible to infections, and that's not fun. Keep oil away from the cooch, and everyone is going to be happier.

This leaves two types of lubrications that are friendly for the vagina. The first is silicone-based. Some well-known brands include Wet

Platinum, Eros Bodyglide, Pjur Bodyglide, Gun Oil (not actually oil based), and Pink. Silicone lube is friendly for the vagina, but isn't compatible with silicone toys, or really any soft, squishy toy. It also, while not poisonous, is not the tastiest of lubes. This might be a great lube to use for manual stimulation prior to, during, or after oral sex (or on its own!), vaginal intercourse, anal stimulation, anal intercourse, hand jobs, and so on. It's also completely compatible with any type of condoms, gloves, and dams.

The second type of lubricant is also the most well-known: water-based lubricant. This is the type of lube that many people think of when they think of store-bought lube. Some well-known vulva-friendly brands include Sliquid, Maximus, Wet Naturals, Pink Water, and Blossom Organics. Water-based lube is compatible with all types of toys, with all types of condoms, gloves, and dams, and with most bodies. But some of the flavored water-based lubricants contain sugar. Never use a lubricant with sugar in it near the vulva—that's basically asking for a yeast infection. Sugary lubes are usually sold for novelty use only and, while great for blow jobs, should be kept away from the vagina and the anus. Another ingredient in many water-based lubes is called glycerin. Glycerin is a safe ingredient overall—it's used in soaps, shampoos, and many other health and beauty products. But many vulvas seem to have a negative reaction to glycerin; in some folks, it can cause itching or an allergic reaction, while others can experience yeast infections or irritation. If you or your partner ever has these sensations after using a water-based lubricant that contains glycerin, try out a glycerin-free option, such as those listed above.

How much lube should you use? As much as you want! Keeping the vulva wet and slippery is the name of the game, so add as much as you'd like. With silicone-based lube, it keeps going and going and going, so you probably won't need to reapply or reactivate. With water-based lube, it can dry up as it gets used. For most people, their first inclination is to add more. The problem with that is the lube may get stickier and stickier, until you're web-slinging around the vulva à la Spiderman. Instead of adding more water-based lube, you can actually reactivate the lube by adding more water. You can do this with spit, by pouring a little water on from a cup, glass, or bottle, by hopping in the shower, or by using a mister or squirt gun: it's up to you and your partner and what turns the two of you on.

Some people think that if flavored lube is a good idea (which it definitely can be), other things can double for this, like chocolate syrup, whipped cream, sweet liqueurs, and so on. The problem is that all these things contain sugar. Again, placing sugar on, near, in, or anywhere around the vulva is an open invitation for a yeast infection. Now, I'm not saying that you absolutely cannot eat an ice cream sundae off of your partner's vulva, but if you want to do so, I'd suggest using a layer of plastic kitchen wrap between the vulva and the sugary concoction. Either that, or be prepared to visit the gynecologist and start a round of antibiotics.

HOT DAM!
Making Safer Sex Sexy

For some reason, there's the thought out there that women who have sex with women don't need to be concerned about safer sex . . . which is total bullcrap. HPV (the human papillomavirus), the STI that causes genital warts and cervical cancer, is the fastest-growing STI among women who have sex with women. Herpes (I and II), gonorrhea, and chlamydia are also transmitted from woman to woman, as are yeast infections, and bacteria that can cause UTIs (urinary tract infections). Basically, you're not magically protected from sexually transmitted infections or other nasty bacteria just because the person you're having sex with happens to have a vulva.

How can you protect yourself? First, chat up your partner. Find out when the last time she got tested was and which STIs she was tested for—lots of doctors don't run a full panel, so it's good to know these details. Make sure you share your own testing history with your partner: it takes two to tango, or transmit, as the case may be. Some medical professionals are still a bit ignorant about women who have sex with women, and some of these professionals have been known to state that lesbians don't need Pap smears or STI tests. If this is what they tell you, you have the choice to either advocate and educate your doctor or to find another one. Don't let your doctor's ignorance be the reason you don't get tested.

Women who have sex with women have a lot of options when it comes to barriers.

One barrier often forgotten by women who are sexing up other women is the infamous condom, because sex toys can transmit STIs and bacteria from one partner to another. If you're going to be sharing a toy, using a condom is a way to create a safety barrier, and it also leads to easier clean up—just toss the condom, rinse the toy, and you're done. Better safe than sorry, and condoms can make safety a lot easier.

For many folks, barriers might not seem very fun or sexy at all. That's okay. There are ways to make them more enjoyable, and as you use them, you get more used to having them in your sex life. One easy trick is to use lube between the barrier and the vulva; that can really help transmit the sensations being provided. Think of it as a safer sex sandwich—vulva, lube, barrier, tongue. Gloves sometimes feel better than skin; the smoothness lets the lube spread around more easily, and there are no patches of rough skin, hang nails, and so on to get caught on delicate vulvar or anal tissue.

Do you have to use dams or barriers? Certainly not—you don't have to do anything. But it's important to be educated on safer sex and sexual health, and to make sure that your partner is as well. STIs like herpes, chlamydia, and gonorrhea can all be transmitted through most sexual activity (including two women getting it on together), and sometimes bacterial infections and allergic reactions can be triggered if the person going down has recently smoked or used other chemicals orally. Knowledge is power; use knowledge to make the best decisions for yourself.

Let's have another quick conversation on the use of sugar and sugary products as part of your sexual experience. Vulvas and vaginas, for the most part, do not enjoy sugar in any form, and that sometimes also extends to products containing glucose and even glycerin. Save the sugar for your sweet talk, and keep it away from the vulva.

LONG LIVE YOUR ADVENTURE

This book has covered a lot, from information about your bodies and how they tick to safer sex practices, tips for communication, the lowdown on lube and sex toys, and of course, the endless list of different positions you might want to try once you get down and dirty together. I hope you learned something and can take that to your next sexual encounter, whether that's tonight, next week, next month, or next year.

If you'd like your partner to read through it as well, that's of course highly encouraged. Consider challenging her to guess your favorite new position you want to try, or perhaps sticky-note a page that you want to make sure she reads and just leave it on her nightstand.

There are three rules I have for making sure you're having good sex: communication is key, lube is love, and you've gotta laugh. So make sure you're getting across what you want to your partner (and are open to hearing the same from her); that you're well stocked with lube to keep things slippery, fun, and of course, pleasurable; and that you're able to laugh when the time is right. It's okay to laugh—it'll boost your endorphins and then when you get back to the sex you were having, your body will be even more primed for pleasure.

Whether you're lesbian, straight, heterosexual, heteroflexible, bisexual, queer, pansexual, homosexual, homoflexible, questioning, or more, you have the right to have the sex you want to be having and the knowledge about your own body and that of your partner. There is no one magical way to have lesbian sex, or for two women to have sex at all. The sex you're having, enjoying, and wanting more of is exactly the type of sex that's right for you right now. So continue to have it, tweak it as needed, learn more about yourself and your partner, and bring your confident, sexy, sex-positive attitude into the world.

Vulva love and vibrator wishes,
Shanna

ABOUT THE AUTHOR

Shanna Katz, M.Ed, ACS, is a queer femme, board-certified sexologist, sexuality educator, and author. From topics like relationship communication skills to nonmonogamy, and oral sex to how sexuality and dis/ability intersect, she talks, writes, and teaches about the huge spectrum of sexuality from both personal and professional perspectives. She's using her master's of sexuality education to provide accessible, open-source sex education to people around the country, and is working hard to bring sex education and positivity to the Southwest as well as online.

A member of many sexuality organizations, and member of the board of two sex-positive nonprofits, Shanna is actively involved in work toward equality and social justice for people of all identities. Teaching classes at colleges and universities is one of her favorite ways to expand horizons. She also loves traveling to speak at conferences, sex toy stores, dungeons, women's groups, LGBTQ centers, art galleries, and more, and copresenting with her partner on looking at privilege in sexuality education and LGBTQ-inclusive medical practices. She has been featured by *Men's Health*, *Cosmo*, *Out Front Colorado*, *Westword*, *Echo*, the *New Times*, *Fox News*, and various radio stations nationwide.

She has written for many sexuality websites, had a sexuality-centric radio show, has had her erotica published in multiple anthologies, and has written multiple books on sexuality. When not blogging, teaching, writing, or tweeting about the oh-so-many interesting and awkward moments in her life, Shanna can be found drinking tea, eating cupcakes, and cuddling with her partner and their three rescued cats. For more info, please visit her sexuality education site, www.ShannaKatz.com. Follow her on Twitter @shanna_katz or friend her at www.Facebook.com/ShannaKatz.

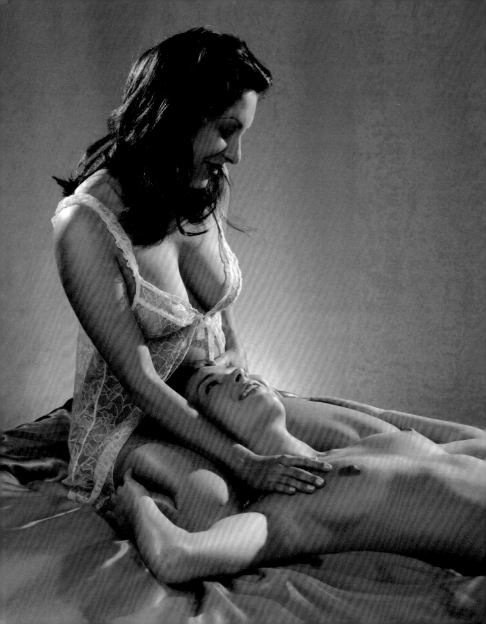